GLOBAL HARMONIZATION OF METHODOLOGICAL APPROACHES TO NUTRIENT INTAKE RECOMMENDATIONS

PROCEEDINGS OF A WORKSHOP

Leslie Pray and Ann L. Yaktine, *Rapporteurs*

Food and Nutrition Board

Health and Medicine Division

The National Academies of
SCIENCES · ENGINEERING · MEDICINE

THE NATIONAL ACADEMIES PRESS
Washington, DC
www.nap.edu

THE NATIONAL ACADEMIES PRESS 500 Fifth Street, NW Washington, DC 20001

This activity was supported by a contract between the National Academy of Sciences and the Bill & Melinda Gates Foundation (#10003263). Any opinions, findings, conclusions, or recommendations expressed in this publication do not necessarily reflect the views of any organization or agency that provided support for the project.

International Standard Book Number-13: 978-0-309-47200-5
International Standard Book Number-10: 0-309-47200-8
Digital Object Identifier: https://doi.org/10.17226/25023

Additional copies of this publication are available for sale from the National Academies Press, 500 Fifth Street, NW, Keck 360, Washington, DC 20001; (800) 624-6242 or (202) 334-3313; http://www.nap.edu.

Printed in the United States of America

Suggested citation: National Academies of Sciences, Engineering, and Medicine. 2018. *Global harmonization of methodological approaches to nutrient intake recommendations: Proceedings of a workshop*. Washington, DC: The National Academies Press. doi: https://doi.org/10.17226/25023.

The National Academies of

SCIENCES • ENGINEERING • MEDICINE

The National Academy of Sciences was established in 1863 by an Act of Congress, signed by President Lincoln, as a private, nongovernmental institution to advise the nation on issues related to science and technology. Members are elected by their peers for outstanding contributions to research. Dr. Marcia McNutt is president.

The National Academy of Engineering was established in 1964 under the charter of the National Academy of Sciences to bring the practices of engineering to advising the nation. Members are elected by their peers for extraordinary contributions to engineering. Dr. C. D. Mote, Jr., is president.

The National Academy of Medicine (formerly the Institute of Medicine) was established in 1970 under the charter of the National Academy of Sciences to advise the nation on medical and health issues. Members are elected by their peers for distinguished contributions to medicine and health. Dr. Victor J. Dzau is president.

The three Academies work together as the **National Academies of Sciences, Engineering, and Medicine** to provide independent, objective analysis and advice to the nation and conduct other activities to solve complex problems and inform public policy decisions. The National Academies also encourage education and research, recognize outstanding contributions to knowledge, and increase public understanding in matters of science, engineering, and medicine.

Learn more about the National Academies of Sciences, Engineering, and Medicine **at www.nationalacademies.org.**

PLANNING COMMITTEE ON THE GLOBAL HARMONIZATION OF METHODOLOGICAL APPROACHES TO NUTRIENT INTAKE RECOMMENDATIONS[1]

STEPHANIE ATKINSON (*Chair*), Professor and Nutrition Clinician-Scientist, Department of Pediatrics, McMaster University
ROSALIND GIBSON, Professor Emerita, Department of Human Nutrition, University of Otago
ANURA KURPAD, Professor and Head, Department of Physiology and Nutrition, St. John's Medical College
SUZANNE MURPHY, Professor Emerita and Researcher, Epidemiology Program, University of Hawaii Cancer Center
JOHN MUYONGA, Professor, Department of Food Technology and Human Nutrition, Makerere University
HEE YOUNG PAIK, Director, Center for Gendered Innovations in Science and Technology Research, Korea Federation of Women's Science and Technology Associations
ANN PRENTICE, Director and Head, Nutrition and Bone Health Research, Medical Research Council Elsie Widdowson Laboratory, University of Cambridge
STANLEY ZLOTKIN, Professor, Pediatrics and Nutritional Sciences, Hospital for Sick Children, University of Toronto

Health and Medicine Division Staff

ANN L. YAKTINE, Study Director
AMANDA NGUYEN, Associate Program Officer
MEREDITH YOUNG, Senior Program Assistant
ANN L. YAKTINE, Director, Food and Nutrition Board

[1] The National Academies of Sciences, Engineering, and Medicine's planning committees are solely responsible for organizing the workshop, identifying topics, and choosing speakers. The responsibility for the published Proceedings of a Workshop rests with the workshop rapporteurs and the institution.

Reviewers

This Proceedings of a Workshop was reviewed in draft form by individuals chosen for their diverse perspectives and technical expertise. The purpose of this independent review is to provide candid and critical comments that will assist the National Academies of Sciences, Engineering, and Medicine in making each published proceedings as sound as possible and to ensure that it meets the institutional standards for quality, objectivity, evidence, and responsiveness to the charge. The review comments and draft manuscript remain confidential to protect the integrity of the process.

We thank the following individuals for their review of this proceedings:

CELINE DUMAS, European Food Safety Authority
VALERIE FRIESEN, Global Alliance for Improved Nutrition
ALICE LICHTENSTEIN, Jean Mayer-U.S. Department of Agriculture (USDA) Human Nutrition Research Center on Aging
SIMIN MEYDANI, Jean Mayer-USDA Human Nutrition Research Center on Aging

Although the reviewers listed above provided many constructive comments and suggestions, they were not asked to endorse the content of the proceedings nor did they see the final draft before its release. The review of this proceedings was overseen by **DIANE BIRT,** Iowa State University. She was responsible for making certain that an independent examination of this proceedings was carried out in accordance with standards of the National Academies and that all review comments were carefully considered. Responsibility for the final content rests entirely with the rapporteurs and the National Academies.

Contents

ACRONYMS AND ABBREVIATIONS xv

1 INTRODUCTION 1
Defining the Problem: Partner Panel, 4
Organization of This Proceedings, 7

2 BACKGROUND FOR THE WORKSHOP 9
Overview, 9
Harmonizing the Nutrient Intake Values: Phase 1, 10
Applications and Uses of Nutrient Intake Recommendations, 17

3 HARMONIZATION FRAMEWORKS 21
Overview, 21
Framework Consultation Process: Key Issues and Conclusions, 23
Endpoints: Differences When Considering Deficiency Versus Chronic Disease, 28
Guiding Principles for Developing Dietary Reference Intakes Based on Chronic Disease: Highlights of the Consensus Report, 35
Discussion, 38

4 CURRENT MODELS FOR ESTABLISHING INTAKE RECOMMENDATIONS 43
Overview, 43
Dietary Reference Intakes: Harmonized Nutrient Standards for Canada and the United States, 45
South Australia and New Zealand, 46
South Korea: 2015 Dietary Reference Intakes for Koreans, 48
United Kingdom, 50
Discussion, 51

5 EXPLORING APPROACHES TO EVALUATING THE EVIDENCE 57
Overview, 57
Tools for Evaluating Strength and Quality of Evidence, 59
Global Systematic Reviews: How Can It Be Done?, 65
Risk–Benefit Assessment of Foods in a European Perspective, 72
Discussion, 79

6 CONTEXTUAL FACTORS: HOST, DIET/ENVIRONMENT, AND HEALTH STATUS 83
Overview, 83
The Role of the Host: Genetic Variation, 86
The Role of the Host: Physiology Adaptation, 93
The Role of Health Status: Infection, 96
The Role of Health Status: Aging, 100
The Role of Diet and Environment in Setting Nutrient Bioavailability Factors for Estimating Dietary Requirements, 105
The Role of Diet on Nutrient Bioavailability: Issues for Habitual Diets of Asian Countries, 110
Discussion, 113

7 BREAKOUT DISCUSSIONS: APPLICATIONS, FACILITATING QUALITY, AND COST-EFFECTIVENESS 117
Overview, 117
Setting the Stage, 118
Question 1: Advantages of Global Harmonization of Methodologies, 120
Question 2: Additional Resources and Expertise to Facilitate Adoption of a Harmonized Approach, 121
Question 3: Likely Barriers and Challenges to Achieving Global Harmonization, 122
Synthesis of Breakout Discussion, 123
Discussion, 124

8 EXPLORING ADVANTAGES, BARRIERS, AND CHALLENGES TO GLOBAL HARMONIZATION OF METHODOLOGIES FOR NUTRIENT INTAKE RECOMMENDATIONS **127**
Overview, 127
EURRECA (European Micronutrient Recommendations Aligned), 130
EFSA (European Food Safety Authority), 132
Africa, 134
Norway, 135
Southeast Asia, 136
Discussion, 138

9 MOVING THE CONVERSATION FORWARD **143**
Chair's Closing Summary, 143
Chair's Three Strategic Messages, 145

REFERENCES **147**

APPENDIXES

A Workshop Agenda 155
B Speaker and Facilitator Biographies 161

Boxes, Figures, and Table

BOXES

1-1 Statement of Task, 2

2-1 Overview of Points Presented by Individual Speakers, 10

3-1 Overview of Points Presented by Individual Speakers, 22

4-1 Overview of Points Presented by Individual Speakers, 44

5-1 Overview of Points Presented by Individual Speakers, 58

6-1 Overview of Points Presented by Individual Speakers, 84

8-1 Overview of Points Presented by Individual Speakers, 128

FIGURES

2-1 Nutrient intake values (NIVs) framework developed by the 2005–2007 international harmonization initiative, 16
2-2 Risk of inadequacy and risk of excess as a function of observed level of intake, 18
2-3 Group-level intake distribution as a function of intake, 18

3-1 Evidence pyramid describing quality of evidence and risk of bias associated with different types of studies, 30
3-2 Risk of inadequacy and risk of adverse effects as a function of observed level of nutrient intake, 32
3-3 Differences in the risks of chronic diseases versus toxicity with increasing nutrient intake levels, 34

5-1 A flow chart of events that occur during a study, with the seven different types of biases that can occur along the way, 60
5-2 The nutrition-specific quality assessment instrument (QAI) developed by Wells and colleagues for Health Canada with the same internal validity checklist as in the original SIGN 50 QAI, plus the newly developed nutrition-specific section and a revised overall assessment section, 63
5-3 Generic analytic framework for a systematic review of studies on the associations between a nutrient and health outcomes, 68
5-4 Analytic framework for vitamin D and/or calcium and associated health outcomes, 69
5-5 Analytic framework for vitamin D and/or calcium and associated safety-related (adverse) outcomes, 70
5-6 Population distribution versus intake for a hypothetical nutrient, 75
5-7 Risk–benefit curve showing risk of effects associated with deficient intake, risk of adverse effects associated with excessive intake, and the lack of risk associated with intake at the safe upper limit, 77

6-1 Maps of lactose tolerance phenotype frequencies and predicted lactose tolerance phenotype frequencies based on lactose tolerance-associated allele frequencies, 89
6-2 The Bayesian model used by WHO (2015a) to develop its new guidelines for red blood cell (RBC) folate concentrations for women of reproductive age, 91
6-3 Dose–response curve computed from the Bayesian model used by WHO (2015a), overlaid with clinical data from Daly et al. (1995), 92

TABLE

5-1 Predicted Public Health Burden (DALYs) Associated with Different Levels of Flour Folic Acid Fortification, 76

Acronyms and Abbreviations

ADI	acceptable daily intake
AHRQ	Agency for Healthcare Research and Quality
AI	adequate intake
AMDR	acceptable macronutrient distribution range
ANR	average nutrient requirement
BMI	body mass index
BMR	basal metabolic rate
CACFP	Child and Adult Care Food Program
CCHS	Canadian Community Health Survey
CNV	copy number variant
CV	coefficient of variation
DALY	disability-adjusted life year
DEXA	dual-energy X-ray absorptiometry
DFE	dietary folate equivalent
DRI	Dietary Reference Intake
DRV	dietary reference value
EAR	estimated average requirement
EFSA	European Food Safety Authority
EPC	Evidence-based Practice Center
EU	European Union
EURRECA	European Micronutrient Recommendations Aligned

FAO	Food and Agriculture Organization
FNB	Food and Nutrition Board
GEMS	Global Environment Monitoring System
GIFT	Global Individual Food consumption data Tool
GRADE	Grading of Recommendations Assessment, Development and Evaluation
HMD	Health and Medicine Division
ICN2	Second International Conference on Nutrition
ILSI	International Life Sciences Institute
INFOODS	International Network of Food Data Systems
INL	individual nutrient level
IOM	Institute of Medicine
IUNS	International Union of Nutritional Sciences
IZiNCG	International Zinc Nutrition Consultative Group
JAMA	*Journal of the American Medical Association*
JPI	Joint Programming Initiative
KNS	Korean Nutrition Society
KRDA	Korean recommended dietary allowance
LDL	low-density lipoprotein
LOAEL	lowest-observed-adverse-effect-level
LRNI	lower reference nutrient intake
NFCS	Nationwide Food Consumption Survey
NHANES	National Health and Nutrition Examination Survey
NHMRC	National Health and Medical Research Council
NIV	nutrient intake value
NOAEL	no-observed-adverse-effect-level
NOFA	nutrients and other food substances
NRV	nutrient reference value
PICOS	population, interventions/exposures, comparators, and outcomes of interest
PUFA	polyunsaturated fatty acid
QAI	quality assessment instrument

RBC	red blood cell
RCT	randomized controlled trial
RDA	recommended dietary allowance
RIVM	Netherlands National Institute for Public Health and the Environment
RNI	reference nutrient intake
SCF	Scientific Committee on Food
SNAP	Supplemental Nutrition Assistance Program
SNP	single nucleotide polymorphism
SRDR	Systematic Review Data Repository
UK	United Kingdom
UL	tolerable upper intake level
UN	United Nations
UNICEF	United Nations Children's Fund
UNL	upper nutrient level
USDA	U.S. Department of Agriculture
UV	ultraviolet
WHO	World Health Organization
WIC	Supplemental Nutrition Program for Women, Infants, and Children

1

Introduction

The Food and Nutrition Board (FNB) of the National Academies of Sciences, Engineering, and Medicine, in partnership with the Department of Nutrition for Health and Development of the World Health Organization (WHO) and the Nutrition Division of the Food and Agriculture Organization (FAO), convened an open public workshop that was available in person and on the web to explore the evidence for achieving global harmonization of methodological approaches to establishing nutrient intake recommendations.[1] The workshop was held at the FAO headquarters in Rome, Italy, September 21–22, 2017. The workshop objectives, guided by the Statement of Task (see Box 1-1) and identified by the workshop planning committee, were the following:

- Describe potential frameworks to enable global harmonization of methodologies to establish nutrient intake recommendations.
- Explore approaches for evaluating the evidence to facilitate global harmonization of methodologies to establish nutrient intake recommendations.
- Examine the potential for addressing contextual factors from different population subgroups, regions, and countries that may or may not be conducive to harmonization.

[1]Throughout this publication, unless otherwise indicated, harmonization refers to the harmonization of methodological approaches to establishing nutrient intake values, not the harmonization of actual values.

BOX 1-1
Statement of Task

The Food and Nutrition Board, in partnership with the Department of Nutrition for Health and Development of the World Health Organization (WHO) and the Nutrition Division of the Food and Agriculture Organization (FAO), will convene an ad hoc committee to plan and organize a workshop to explore questions about the uses of nutrient intake recommendations, the frameworks used for their development, the status of nutrient intake recommendations globally, and experiences and expertise in methodological approaches. The workshop is intended to review current nutrient intake recommendations; discuss the feasibility of harmonizing approaches to setting such recommendations globally; examine the development of principles by which they may be applied in diverse contexts that relate to individuals or populations, or regulatory purposes; and examine perceptions and acceptance of nutrient intake recommendations by different stakeholders. The goal is to develop discussion topics about ways to provide a uniform and consistent basis for setting nutrient intake recommendations across countries while accommodating culturally and context-specific food choices and dietary patterns.

Specific issues for consideration can include

- Identifying appropriate uses for and ways to reach consensus on nutrient intake standards;
- Developing a harmonized framework and approaches for the derivation of nutrient intake recommendations;
- Cultivating international partnerships to evaluate methodologies and approaches to reviewing nutrients;
- Reviewing the process for harmonization approaches and development of nutrient intake recommendations to maximize their acceptance;

- Consider approaches to facilitate global sharing of resources to maintain quality and support cost-effectiveness to develop methodologies for nutrient intake recommendations.
- Identify the advantages, barriers, and challenges to global harmonization of methodologies to establish nutrient intake recommendations.

In his welcoming remarks, Kostas Stamoulis, assistant director-general of FAO's Economic and Social Development Department, described nutrition as a fundamental pillar of FAO work. "The nutrition community has been sounding the alarm for a long time," he said. Now, with one in three people on earth suffering from some form of malnutrition (i.e., undernutrition, critical nutrition deficiency, overweight, or obesity) and caught in a vicious cycle of malnutrition and poverty, the international community has taken notice. In 2014, United Nations (UN) member states gathered

- Reviewing criteria and approaches for establishing priorities for nutrient reviews;
- Suggesting processes for incorporating different contextual issues and addressing differences across regions and countries, including but not limited to, documenting case studies;
- Undertaking evidence reviews on topics related to setting acceptable recommendations;
- Reviewing mechanisms for performing and/or evaluating nutrient reviews;
- Assuring accessibility to data across global partners;
- Maintaining cost-effectiveness by:
  - Using cost-effective approaches that do not compromise on quality;
  - Sharing cost across global partners to reduce the burden to any single country and/or international agency; and
  - Establishing consistency in approaches to reduce the overall cost burden;
- Discussing options for further examination of a selected nutrient of global public health concern for which there is substantive and significant disagreement on current reference values.

The planning committee will use the discussion topics it develops as a basis for planning a 2–3 day workshop to discuss the uses, status, and development of nutrient intake recommendations globally; provide a venue for sharing information on methodological approaches and potential international processes for the development and standardization of nutrient intake recommendations; and examine the perception and acceptance of these values in a global setting. The planning committee will identify the topics to be addressed, develop the agenda, and select and invite speakers. A brief summary and a full-length summary of the workshop proceedings will be prepared by a rapporteur, reviewed, and published in accordance with institutional guidelines.

at the Second International Conference on Nutrition (ICN2) and committed to eradicate hunger and prevent all forms of malnutrition. The 2030 Agenda for Sustainable Development reiterated the need to end malnutrition in all its forms, with Goal 2 being to end hunger, achieve food security and improved nutrition, and promote sustainable agriculture. Then, the UN General Assembly declared, in April 2016, the period between 2016 through 2025 the "UN decade of nutrition." Together, these three actions, along with numerous regional declarations to promote nutrition "have placed nutrition firmly at the heart of the development debate," Stamoulis said. The development agenda recognizes firmly that transformed food systems, not just agriculture, have a fundamental role to play in promoting healthy diets and improving nutrition.

The challenge for FAO as an organization, as Stamoulis suspected was true for many organizations, is how to turn this political commitment into action at the country level. Over its first 50 years, FAO worked very closely in collaboration with WHO to continuously support the provision of scientific advice on nutrient requirements to member countries and international bodies. However, despite all of this work, there is little consistency in the approaches used to set country-level nutrient intake recommendations. Moreover, there are few processes in place to ensure that these recommendations are properly updated and remain relevant to target population groups. In this regard, Stamoulis concluded, FAO looked forward to the outcomes of this workshop.

For Stephanie Atkinson, McMaster University professor of pediatrics and chair of the workshop planning committee, this workshop has been an outcome of a nearly 25-year journey. In 1995, Atkinson was the Canadian representative to the oversight committee for the first harmonization of Dietary Reference Intakes (DRIs) between Canada and the United States. In 1997, Canada hosted the International Union of Nutritional Sciences (IUNS) International Congress in Montreal, where an informal luncheon was held to talk about harmonization of the Canadian and U.S. DRIs. Atkinson noted that several people in attendance at the workshop had also attended that 1997 luncheon. People were interested, but a little apprehensive, Atkinson recalled. But they did develop, over the next 10 years, harmonized DRIs for the two countries. Then, in 2005, the UN University's Food and Nutrition Programme, in collaboration with FAO, WHO, and the UN Children's Fund (UNICEF), sponsored an international harmonization initiative, led by Janet King and Cutberto Garza. "That was, we thought, the next big step," Atkinson said. She noted that King would be describing the work later during the workshop (a summary of King's presentation is provided in Chapter 2). Her hope was that it would not be another 10 years before reaching consensus and realizing a globally implementable plan for harmonization of methodological approaches to setting nutrient-based recommendations.

DEFINING THE PROBLEM: PARTNER PANEL

Following Stamoulis's and Atkinson's welcoming remarks, representatives from WHO and FAO were invited to offer further opening remarks in the first panel of the workshop: "Defining the Problem: Partner Panel." Atkinson spoke on the behalf of Ken Brown of the Bill & Melinda Gates Foundation.

WHO

Like Atkinson, Chizuru Nishida, WHO coordinator of the Nutrition Policy and Scientific Advice Unit in the Department of Nutrition for Health and Development, viewed this workshop as an opportunity to build on the 2005–2007 initiative, including the 10 commissioned background review papers, each on a specific aspect of the process for harmonizing nutrient intake values (NIVs). She repeated that the focus of that initiative was not on the values themselves (i.e., NIVs) but on how to harmonize the concepts and approaches for developing them.

At around that same time, Nishida recalled, as requested by WHO's World Health Assembly, some transformations were being implemented in the way WHO guidelines were developed. Specifically, in 2007, the Guidelines Review Committee was set up to harmonize guidelines across all WHO program areas, including in diet and nutrition, and to ensure that WHO guidelines were consistent with internationally accepted best practices, based on evidence through systematic reviews where appropriate, and based on a transparent process for evaluating the quality of evidence and strength of recommendations. WHO began implementing this new harmonized approach for guideline development throughout its organization in January 2009, with mandatory implementation initiated in January 2010.

Additionally, as part of its efforts to strengthen its scientific advice on nutrition, WHO proposed to establish a global network of institutions for scientific advice on nutrition, initially by bringing together public institutions involved in developing national diet- and nutrition-related guidelines to explore the possibility of facilitating synergy and avoiding replication of work. In March 2010, WHO held the first face-to-face meeting of this global network in Geneva (WHO, 2010). The objective of the meeting was to share information and to learn about each other's ongoing and planned work. Through this network, Nishida explained, WHO hopes to explore whether there is a way to harmonize how evidence is extracted so it can be shared and used collectively among public institutions, including international, normative agencies like WHO and FAO. The outcome of the 2010 meeting indicated, according to Nishida, that although everyone was willing to collaborate and harmonize, they viewed implementation as difficult. Thus, there was hesitation to move forward.

Since then, however, nearly 10 years have passed. She expressed hope that this work will not just further the discussion,[2] but will provide a road map of possible next steps for facilitating global harmonization, including the identification of priority nutrients or areas where proposed approaches can be tested. Additionally, she expressed WHO's interest in the possibility of applying or incorporating existing processes and methodologies already

[2] This workshop will help to inform a larger, consensus effort to review and assess methodological approaches to developing nutrient intake recommendations, as described at http://nationalacademies.org/hmd/Activities/Nutrition/NutrientIntakeRecommendations.aspx (accessed April 25, 2018).

in use by different agencies and institutions, such as those being implemented by WHO (e.g., the organization-wide effort to harmonize guideline development).

Food and Agriculture Organization (FAO) of the United Nations

Anna Lartey, FAO director of nutrition, began her remarks by mentioning that she attended the 1997 IUNS International Congress in Montreal, which Atkinson had mentioned. At the time, she was a graduate student at the University of California, Davis, unaware that one day she would become president of IUNS. Her term would end in October 2017, she noted. Also in October, FAO would turn 72 years old. Yet, the mandates that resulted in establishment of FAO remain, she said, and remain to be relevant. This includes raising the level of nutrition of the people under FAO's jurisdiction.

Lartey then described some of FAO's ongoing programs in nutrition that are relevant to work on the harmonization of methodological approaches to developing nutrient intake recommendations, noting FAO's emphasis over the past 5 years on reforming food systems to deliver healthy diets. "We believe that if we want to address all forms of malnutrition as we currently have it," she said, "we really have to look at sustainable food systems."

First, she mentioned FAO's collaboration with WHO to develop the Global Individual Food consumption data Tool (GIFT), a dynamic platform for capturing individual food consumption data (FAO/WHO, 2017). By providing age and sex disaggregated data on individual food consumption, GIFT will help to answer the question, what are people eating? She explained that when individual or household food consumption data and food composition data are converted into energy and nutrients, they can be compared to recommended nutrient intake references. Another relevant FAO activity is its work over the past year to organize trainings for over 24 Anglophone and Francophone countries to support these countries in developing and implementing national food-based dietary guidelines. Also relevant, in 2014, FAO and partners developed a minimum dietary diversity score for women to use as a global indicator for assessing women's diet quality. Now, with the support of the European Union, FAO is supporting countries to include this indicator in their country-monitoring frameworks.

One of the inefficiencies in food systems, Lartey continued, is the huge loss and waste of food. FAO estimates that about one-third of the food produced for human consumption becomes food waste or is lost somewhere along the value chain. To address this, FAO, as custodian of Sustainable Development Goal 2, which Stamoulis described previously, has agreed to develop a global indicator against which countries can report on their food loss and waste using a common methodology.

FAO is interested not only in what people are eating, but also in whether they are meeting their nutrient requirements for optimal health and nutrition. However, many member states, especially those in the developing world, do not have the resources and technical capacity to develop their own national recommended nutrient intakes and, as such, they depend on WHO and FAO for guidance. Lartey expects this work to be very useful in continuing to guide other countries in the development of nutrient intake tables. She concluded by echoing calls to put harmonization "into action," particularly as the UN has declared this next decade the decade of action on nutrition. "Let's give [countries that do not have nutrient intake tables] some basis around which they can determine some of these figures for their own countries," she said.

Bill & Melinda Gates Foundation

To conclude this opening Partner Panel, Atkinson spoke on the behalf of Ken Brown of the Bill & Melinda Gates Foundation, which provided a generous grant for the workshop. According to Brown, as conveyed by Atkinson, the Gates Foundation will judge this effort as being successful if the consensus group,[3] not this workshop, is able to develop recommendations for a preferred method to approach global harmonization and apply this method to the derivation of nutrient intakes for one or more nutrients as an example. Brown also remarked, again, as conveyed by Atkinson, that the Gates Foundation recognizes that the process of global harmonization will require not only technical considerations, but political consensus on how best to apply the recommended approach and which organization or organizations should take the lead on implementing the consensus committee's recommendations.

ORGANIZATION OF THIS PROCEEDINGS

The organization of this Proceedings of a Workshop parallels the organization of the workshop (see Appendix A for the workshop agenda). This introductory chapter summarizes the statement of task, welcoming remarks, and the first panel of the workshop. Chapter 2 summarizes the

[3] The consensus group, separate from the planning committee for this workshop, will be using the evidence presented and the discussions that took place here to review and assess methodological approaches to developing nutrient intake recommendations. Information on the consensus study, including other relevant meetings, is available at http://nationalacademies.org/hmd/Activities/Nutrition/NutrientIntakeRecommendations.aspx (accessed April 25, 2018).

"Background for the Workshop" section of the workshop agenda, which included two presentations, one by Janet King, the second by Suzanne Murphy. Chapter 3 summarizes the first part of session 1, "Harmonization Frameworks," which included a presentation on harmonization efforts in Australia and two presentations on the harmonized U.S.–Canadian approach to setting nutrient reference values for chronic disease. The remainder of session 1, which was a panel discussion, "Current Models for Establishing Intake Recommendations," with four panelists from different regions of the world discussing opportunities for and challenges of harmonization, is summarized in Chapter 4. Chapter 5 summarizes the session 2 presentations on "Approaches to Evaluating the Evidence," with three presentations on quality assessment instruments, systematic reviews, and risk–benefit analysis. Chapter 6 summarizes session 3, "Contextual Factors: Host, Diet/Environment, and Health Status," with a total of six presentations covering genetic variation, host physiology, infection, aging, and bioavailability, and their effects on nutrient intake values. Chapter 7 summarizes the session 4 breakout discussions on "Applications, Facilitating Quality, and Cost-Effectiveness." The workshop was split into six smaller breakout sessions, with each group assigned one of three questions to consider. Chapter 8 summarizes the session 5 panel discussion on "Advantages, Barriers, and Challenges to Global Harmonization of Methodologies for Nutrient Intake Recommendations." Five panelists, again from different regions of the world, shared their experiences and insights. Finally, Chapter 9 summarizes Atkinson's summary of the workshop and discussion of next steps.

It is important to note that this Proceedings of a Workshop summarizes information presented and discussed at the workshop and is not intended to serve as a comprehensive overview of the subject. Nor are the citations herein intended to serve as a comprehensive set of references for any topic; only references cited on speaker slides or in the workshop briefing notebook are included. Additionally, the information presented here reflects the knowledge and opinions of individual workshop participants and should not be construed as consensus on the part of the workshop planning committee, the FNB, or the National Academies.

2

Background for the Workshop

OVERVIEW

The opening session was moderated by workshop planning committee chair Stephanie Atkinson and provided background information for the workshop. Janet King provided an overview of concepts put together by the 2005 international harmonization initiative. That initiative encompassed not only the actual meeting in Florence, Italy, in 2005, but also publication of 10 commissioned background review papers in *Food and Nutrition Bulletin* in 2007 (King and Garza, 2007). The Florence group developed a new term, nutrient intake value (NIV), but emphasized that NIV is analogous to other terms used around the world (e.g., Dietary Reference Intake [DRI], dietary reference value [DRV]). The Florence group then developed separate frameworks (i.e., factors and criteria to consider) for estimating two NIVs in particular: average nutrient requirement (ANR), also known as estimated average requirement (EAR), and upper nutrient level (UNL), more commonly known as tolerable upper intake level (UL). King described several other issues addressed by the group as well, such as criteria for indicators to use when developing NIVs.

Suzanne Murphy continued where King left off, that is, how an NIV, once established using a globally harmonized methodology, can be used or applied at a country or region level. She reviewed in detail the many critical health applications that depend on accurate nutrient intake recommendations, one of which, the setting of global nutrient standards, was, she said, "the reason we are here today." She added that, while many of the other applications are country specific (e.g., designing food assistance programs), an

BOX 2-1
Overview of Points Presented by Individual Speakers

- Phase 1 of harmonizing the process for developing nutrient intake values, which was the 2005 international harmonization initiative, is the starting point for this workshop (King). The 2005 initiative involved lengthy debate about why to harmonize, as well as which terms to harmonize, with participants finally settling on two, estimated average requirement (EAR) and upper nutrient level (UNL; also known as the tolerable upper nutrient intake level, or UL). The initiative developed separate frameworks for each (King).
- An often overlooked advantage of the harmonization of methods used to assess and plan nutrient intakes for individuals and populations is an increased understanding and more appropriate application of nutrient intake recommendations (Murphy).

often overlooked advantage of harmonization is an increased understanding of these other applications.

This chapter summarizes in detail these two presentations, with an overview of points in Box 2-1.

HARMONIZING THE NUTRIENT INTAKE VALUES: PHASE 1[1]

What Janet King referred to as "phase 1" of harmonizing the process for developing nutrient intake values began in 2005 at a meeting in Florence where 17 scientists convened to review harmonizing approaches for developing nutrient-based dietary intake standards. Phase 1 extended through 2007, when 10 commissioned background review papers were published in the *Food and Nutrition Bulletin* (King and Garza, 2007). King recognized the several individuals, in addition to herself, who were present at this Rome workshop and who were also part of the Florence meeting (i.e., Lindsay Allen, Stephanie Atkinson, Rosalind Gibson, Suzanne Murphy, and Patrick Stover). She then went on to review the concepts that were put together at the Florence meeting and described in detail in the commissioned papers.

Why Harmonize the Process for Developing NIVs?

The 2005 Florence group identified four strategic reasons for harmonization:

[1] This section summarizes information presented by Janet King, Ph.D., senior scientist, Children's Hospital Oakland Research Institute, Oakland, California.

1. improve objectivity and transparency of values developed by different groups;
2. provide a common basis for various NIVs;
3. allow low-income countries, with limited resources, to convene groups for modifying the standards for their specific food supplies or national policies; and
4. provide a common basis across countries and regions for establishing global nutrition policies (i.e., fortification policies, regulatory issues).

King commented that, while these four reasons may seem obvious now, in fact it took the Florence attendees quite a while to pull them together.

Terms to Harmonize

The discussion around which terms to harmonize was very long as well, King recalled. First, they had to decide what they were going to call the values. They finally agreed on *nutrient intake values*, or NIVs, as the term to use when referring to nutrient intake recommendations. They emphasized, however, that NIV is analogous to values already in use in different regions around the world, such as DRI, DRV, and nutrient reference value (NRV).

The "next big debate," King continued, was which aspects of the NIVs to develop. The Florence group decided to develop only two: (1) ANR, which King noted some people call the EAR, and (2) UNL, also known as the UL. The ANR is the midpoint of the range of requirements that exist in a population. Other nutrient values, like the lower reference nutrient intake (LRNI) and recommended dietary allowance (RDA), can be derived from the ANR.

The group agreed, however, that it may not always be possible to develop an ANR and a UNL for all nutrients. In cases where data are not sufficient to develop specific recommendations, it may be necessary to establish a safe or adequate intake (AI) instead.

Framework for Estimating ANRs

The Florence group developed the following framework for establishing ANRs, King described:

- The ANR should be based on the mean intake of a population for a specific nutrient. If those values are not distributed normally, then the data should be normalized and the median value used instead.
- ANRs should be established for all essential nutrients and food components that have public health relevance. In other words,

King said, the group felt that ANRs should be established for fiber, for example, because even though it is not an essential nutrient, it is a food component that has public health relevance.

- The group suggested that acceptable macronutrient distribution ranges be established for carbohydrates, protein, and fat, and that these ranges should be for reducing chronic disease risk associated with the intake of these macronutrients. King emphasized, though, ANRs should be set for protein also because it is an essential nutrient.
- The group felt it was important to consider nutrient–nutrient interactions, such as protein–energy interactions (i.e., as energy intake increases, dietary requirements for protein can decline because the protein is no longer used for energy needs) and vitamin E–polyunsaturated fatty acid (PUFA) relationships. These should be characterized quantitatively, if possible.
- Additionally, it is important to consider subpopulations with special needs, such as smokers and their vitamin C requirements, keeping in mind, however, that ANRs are for apparently healthy individuals.

Framework for Estimating Upper Nutrient Levels (UNLs)

The group developed a separate framework for estimating UNLs:

- A UNL is the highest level of a habitual nutrient intake that possesses no risk of adverse health effects in almost all individuals in the general population.
- UNLs can be determined by applying an uncertainty factor to the no-observed-adverse-effect-level (NOAEL) or lowest-observed-adverse-effect-level (LOAEL), but the magnitude of the uncertainty factors need to be considered on a case-by-case basis. In other words, King explained, it cannot be assumed that the uncertainty factor is the same for all nutrients. "We spent a long time on this particular issue," she recalled.
- The group suggested that uncertainty factors be estimated from a list of potential effects of excessive intakes available in the literature.
- "But what we really need," King continued, are biomarkers that anticipate adverse effects associated with higher levels of nutrient intakes.
- Dose–response data for determining UNLs are limited, especially among pregnant and lactating women, children, and the elderly.

After describing these components of the framework for estimating UNLs, King remarked that there are many research issues that still need to be addressed to fully develop these concepts.

Criteria for Selecting NIV Indicators

Selecting an indicator for an average nutrient recommendation is a challenge, King continued. The Florence group came up with several criteria for selecting NIV indicators:

- There should be a demonstrated dose–response function. In other words, King explained, there should be an observed change in the response of the indicator as intake changes.
- The indicator should be responsive to inadequate or excessive intakes of a single nutrient.
- It should be resistant to rapid daily changes in the response to inadequate, adequate, or excessive intakes. For example, when an individual takes a high dose of vitamin C, their urinary ascorbic acid levels change quite quickly. Thus, urinary ascorbic acid levels would not be an acceptable indicator; they change too quickly and do not reflect the tissue use of vitamin C.
- It needs to be easily measured or accessible with noninvasive methods. Blood samples, for example, would be fine, but tissue biopsies would not be considered noninvasive.
- It should not be responsive to environmental changes other than nutrient intake from all sources. For example, smog should not influence the indicator.

The group recommended that there be a single outcome measure for each nutrient and age group. In other words, King explained, with zinc, for example, use a single indicator, such as plasma zinc level, and do not try to also use a biomarker of inflammation as well. Using more than one outcome measure, she said, "would make the whole process very complicated and probably unwieldy." Additionally, because an NIV will vary with population and outcome, it was recommended that the basis of an NIV be fully described, including how the indicator was selected.

Bioequivalence

According to King, in its discussion of bioavailability, the Florence group developed a concept they called bioequivalence. King remarked that she had not seen the concept used much since the 2007 publication and was unsure if that was because the concept was not readily understood or because it was not needed. Nonetheless, she said, the group did spend some time discussing it and decided that bioequivalence of a nutrient can involve bioavailability or bioefficiency.

They defined bioavailability as it is typically defined, King explained: the proportion of the ingested nutrient absorbed and used through normal metabolic pathways. Because bioavailability is influenced by dietary and host-related factors, the group spent a lot of time, she recalled, thinking about the bioavailability of zinc, calcium, iron, retinol, and folate in particular. The bioavailabilities of all of these nutrients are influenced by the amount of nutrient in the diet, as well as whether an individual is growing, if a woman is pregnant, and other host-related factors.

King explained that they defined bioefficiency as the efficiency with which ingested nutrients, such as the carotenoids and various tocopherols, are absorbed and converted to active forms.

Multiple physiological and food factors can influence bioequivalence, the Florence group recognized. These include enhancers or inhibitors of absorption; differences in efficiency of the metabolic conversions that occur for the carotenoids and the tocopherols; and food processing, treatment, and preparation. King added that the group also spent some time thinking about how infection in an individual, and how nutrient–nutrient interactions, can influence bioequivalence.

Life-Stage Factors

They also addressed various life-stage factors, King continued, again with many long discussions beginning with how to set life-stage groups. For example, should it be done by age? King mentioned that many people are now setting life-stage groups by age (e.g., 0–12 months of age, 1–3 years, 3–6 years, and so on). But should it be done by function instead, for example, whether a child is growing at a certain rate or not? Or, should it be done by potential purposes, that is, by the age at which a child is receiving complementary foods, such as from 6 to 36 months?

Regardless of how life-stage groups are set, the same life-stage groups should be used for all nutrients, the Florence group emphasized. For example, there cannot be one set of life-stage groups for vitamin A and another for folate. "This would make it virtually impossible to apply the values," King said. "So we have to decide on how they are going to be and then use it for all of the nutrients."

They chose to treat pregnancy and lactation as two distinct groups. In other words, King said, do not break down pregnancy into trimesters and make different recommendations for the first, second, and third trimesters. "This would be very difficult to implement," King said, "and, frankly, the physiology of pregnancy alters the utilization of nutrients, so we are not convinced that we really need to make different recommendations for the trimester."

Finally, after spending some time talking about how to derive standard weights and heights for a population, they decided to use the WHO growth standards for infants and children. Additionally, they decided to use the average weight of men and women at 18 years of age throughout the adult years, or, in other words, King said, not to allow "an increase in body weight with age." She remarked that this decision seemed appropriate 10 years ago. But today, given how common it is for adults to gain weight after 18 years of age, she said, "I'm not sure we might see it the same way."

Other Considerations

King described two additional sets of issues that were deliberated at the Florence meeting. The first pertained to extrapolation methods and how to extrapolate from one life-stage group to another when data are lacking. "There is no correct way to do this," she said. "It has to be done on an individual nutrient basis. But what is really important is transparency." Regardless of the method used, it needs to be fully explained. Often it is done by body size or the weight or metabolic weight of an individual. Or, it can be done by energy intake. Or, factorial estimates for growth or milk production during lactation can be used.

Additionally, King and colleagues spent some time thinking about genetic variation in NIVs and agreed that it is very important to consider the prevalence of genetic variation, as well as the penetrance of that variation within a population. The group concluded that it is unlikely that gene–gene interactions will affect NIVs because of the low prevalence associated with highly penetrant genes. Additionally, the group considered whether or not there might be gene variants that are linked to nutrient sensitivity (e.g., salt sensitivity), although they did not come up with any conclusions. King commented on how much this area of research has expanded in the past 10 years and that Patrick Stover would be providing an update in his presentation (Stover's presentation is summarized in Chapter 6).

NIV Framework

The NIV framework developed by King and colleagues at the 2005 Florence meeting is illustrated in Figure 2-1. The committee focused most of its attention on the two left columns, King noted.

As illustrated in the middle column of Figure 2-1, the group decided to make recommendations for only two types of values: ANR and UNL. However, it recognized that one can also derive an individual nutrient level (INL) from the ANR, often by extrapolating from the ANR up to a higher

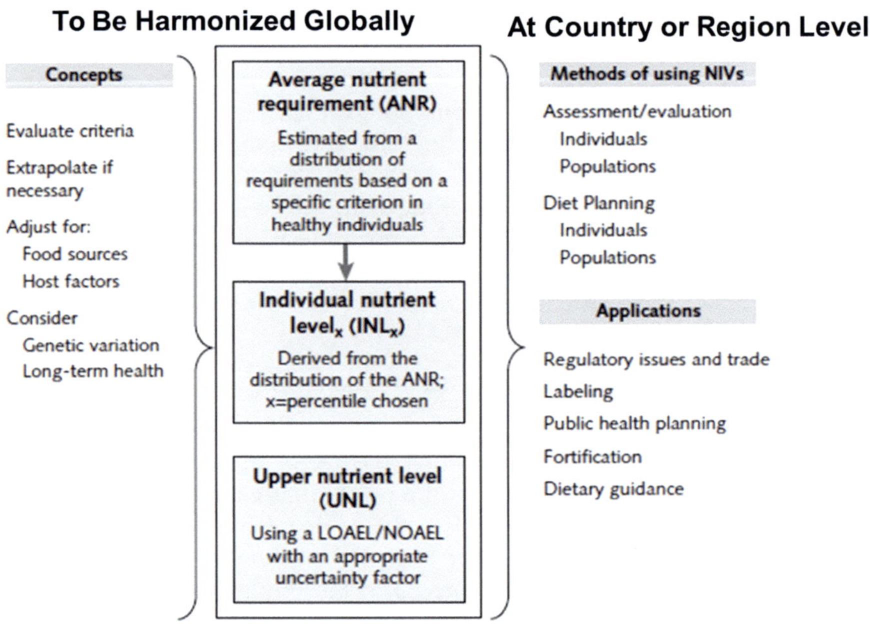

FIGURE 2-1 Nutrient intake values (NIVs) framework developed by the 2005–2007 international harmonization initiative.
NOTE: LOAEL = lowest-observed-adverse-effect-level; NOAEL = no-observed-adverse-effect-level.
SOURCES: Presented by Janet King, HMD Workshop, Rome, Italy, September 21, 2017 (King and Garza, 2007; reprinted by permission of SAGE Publications, Inc.).

level (e.g., 95 percent of the population, 97.5 percent, or even 85 percent if a committee so chooses).

The concepts that serve as the basis of these recommendations include (i.e., left column in Figure 2-1): having a clear understanding of the criteria for the recommendations, how to extrapolate if necessary, how to make adjustments for differences in food sources and host health, and whether there is a need to consider genetic variation or long-term health.

The right column in Figure 2-1 lists other aspects that the committee felt need to be considered at the country or region level, specifically how to use NIVs for assessing or evaluating the adequacy of nutrient intakes in individuals or populations and how to plan diets for individuals and populations. King noted that Suzanne Murphy would be discussing these and the other applications of NIVs in more detail (the summary of Murphy's presentation follows).

APPLICATIONS AND USES OF NUTRIENT INTAKE RECOMMENDATIONS[2]

Suzanne Murphy provided an overview of the uses of nutrient intake recommendations to assess and plan intakes for both individuals and populations; she also reviewed the many critical health applications that depend on accurate nutrient intake recommendations.

She began by emphasizing the importance of using the paradigm illustrated in Figure 2-2. For individuals, intake should be between the recommended INL and the UNL that is not likely to pose a risk of adverse effects. For groups, most people should have intakes between the ANR and UNL (see Figure 2-3).

This paradigm and its methods for evaluating individual and group intakes can be applied to four categories of health applications, Murphy explained: (1) assessment applications for individuals, including evaluating a person's diet; (2) planning applications for individuals, such as offering dietary advice; (3) assessment applications for groups, including evaluating dietary surveys; and (4) planning applications for groups, including designing food fortification programs.

To explain the importance of nutrient standards to policy makers, government agencies, and others, collaborators in the United States and Canada spent about 2 years, Murphy said, developing a two-sided handout listing 10 critical health applications that depend on nutrient standards. While developed for the United States and Canada, the list is universally applicable, in Murphy's opinion. She described each application:

1. Food-based dietary guidelines: Most countries have these, Murphy noted. Examples include the U.S. *Dietary Guidelines for Americans*, U.S. Department of Agriculture (USDA) Food Patterns, and Canada's Food Guide. WHO, FAO, and others have communicated the importance of considering nutrient priorities when developing food-based guidelines (FAO/WHO, 1998). Yet, Murphy said, "you'd be surprised how many people in the United States don't recognize that link."
2. Nutrition monitoring: Examples include the U.S. National Health and Nutrition Examination Survey (NHANES) and the Canadian Community Health Survey (CCHS). Without nutrient standards, Murphy said, it would be impossible to assess nutrient adequacy in the country based on food intake surveys. Both household- and individual-level surveys can be used to examine the prevalence

[2] This section summarizes information presented by Suzanne Murphy, Ph.D., R.D., professor emerita and researcher, University of Hawaii, Honolulu, Hawaii.

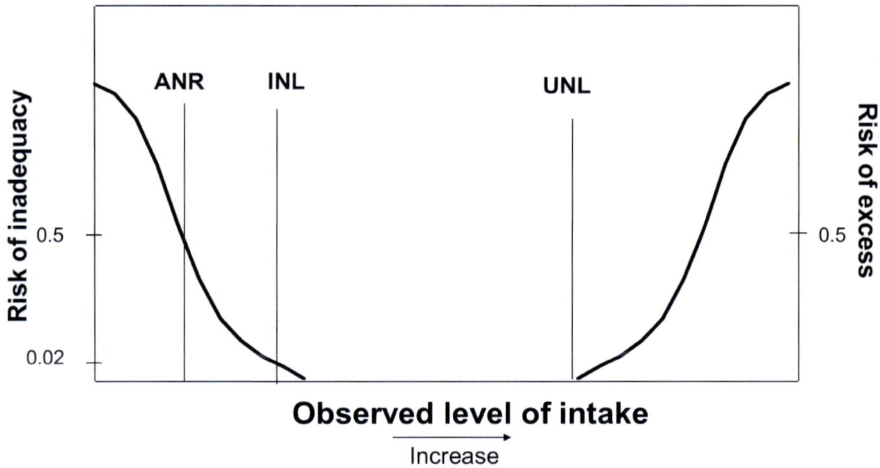

FIGURE 2-2 Risk of inadequacy (left y-axis) and risk of excess (right y-axis) as a function of observed level of intake (x-axis).
NOTE: ANR = average nutrient level; INL = individual nutrient level; UNL = upper nutrient level.
SOURCE: Presented by Suzanne Murphy, HMD Meeting, Rome, Italy, September 22, 2017 (reprinted with permission).

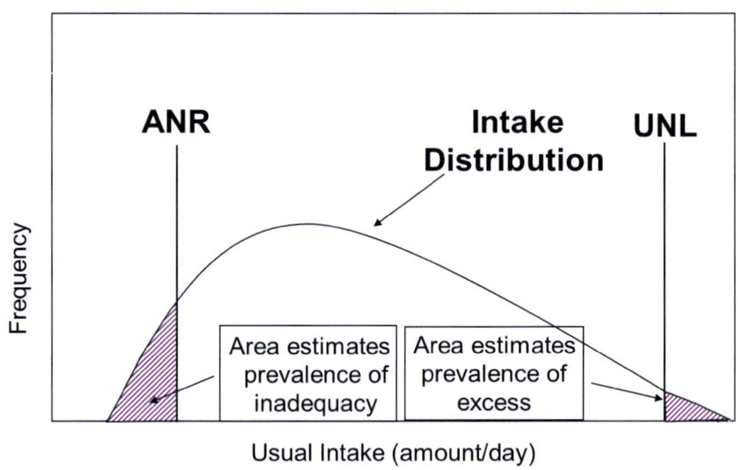

FIGURE 2-3 Group-level intake distribution as a function of intake.
NOTE: ANR = average nutrient requirement; UNL = upper nutrient level.
SOURCE: Presented by Suzanne Murphy, HMD Meeting, Rome, Italy, September 22, 2017 (reprinted with permission).

of inadequacies. She showed a NHANES (2001–2002) bar chart illustrating the prevalence of inadequacy of nutrients in the United States, Although vitamin E tops the list, its inadequacy prevalence (93 percent) is controversial, Murphy said, and can probably be disregarded. However, the others, in her opinion, are more reasonable and allow policy makers to decide where to focus their efforts: second to vitamin E is magnesium, at 56 percent inadequacy, followed by vitamin A at 44 percent; vitamin C at 31 percent; vitamin B6 at 14 percent; zinc at 12 percent; folate at 8 percent; copper, phosphorous, and thiamin all at 5 percent; iron at 4 percent; protein at 3 percent, and carbohydrate, selenium, niacin, and riboflavin all at less than 3 percent.

3. Food assistance programs: Many programs depend on nutrient standards to design their food aid, Murphy said, including school meal programs, the Special Supplemental Nutrition Program for Women, Infants, and Children (WIC), the Supplemental Nutrition Assistance Program (SNAP), and the Child and Adult Care Food Program (CACFP), as well as Administration on Aging programs.
4. Health professionals: Health professionals use nutrient standards for dietary counseling and education and to design diets for groups of people (e.g., in hospitals, prisons, long-term care).
5. Nutrition research: Knowledge of nutrient requirements contributes to the study of how diet helps to prevent disease. Additionally, Murphy said, knowing where data on nutrient requirements are missing provides a frame of reference for research. She noted that harmonization would have an effect on the latter application in particular (i.e., by helping to identify missing data on requirements).
6. Nutrition labeling: This too, Murphy said, is a very global application (see item 10).
7. Military: Murphy mentioned a past committee on military nutrition that not only used nutrient standards but also developed their own in some cases. Nutrient standards remain important for the military for numerous applications, she said.
8. Food and supplement industries: These industries can use nutrient standards to develop healthy foods and safe supplements, Murphy said.
9. Food policies: This includes policies at many levels of government, Murphy noted, and also at schools.
10. Global nutrient standards: Providing a framework for nutrient standards is "why we are here today," Murphy said. A global approach to setting nutrient standards has many potential applications such as assisting the Codex Alimentarius Commission in setting its standards and recommendations, establishing interna-

tional fortification policies, and promoting trade by standardizing nutrition labeling.

In conclusion, Murphy stated that it is possible to harmonize methods used to assess and plan intakes for individuals and populations. Although many of the applications she listed depend on country-specific guidelines, she said, "We can still learn a great deal by sharing our experiences."

Finally, Murphy listed several advantages of harmonization. These include less redundancy (i.e., more efficient use of professional time), the pooling of limited funds so there is no large burden on any specific country or region, a more timely update process so out-of-date values will not lead to inappropriate policies, and increased understanding of uses and more appropriate applications of recommendations. She noted that this last advantage is an often overlooked one.

3

Harmonization Frameworks

OVERVIEW

In session 1, moderated by Peter Clifton, three speakers offered a sketch of the harmonization work completed since the 2005 initiative. This chapter summarizes these presentations and the discussion that followed, with strategic points highlighted here and in Box 3-1.

First, Clifton described consulting work he was involved with in Australia regarding which existing (2005–2006) nutrient reference values (NRVs) to review (i.e., all or some) and how the review process should occur. The existing NRV process had followed the Institute of Medicine (IOM) recommendations almost completely, Clifton recalled, but the process had generated considerable confusion because of its lack of transparency. Among other recommendations for future NRV revisions, the consultative group called for greater transparency in the decision-making process, including clear justification for the inclusion of experts on committees and clear documentation of the process of determining nutrient values.

Next, Amanda MacFarlane discussed the challenges of developing Dietary Reference Intakes (DRIs) based on chronic disease endpoints, as opposed to traditional nutrient deficiency (or excess) endpoints. She explained how risk assessment is at the heart of the DRI framework, but that several critical assumptions of this approach, such as causality, do not always fit for chronic disease endpoints. Causality relies heavily on randomized controlled trials (RCTs), she said, yet most data comparing nutrient intake and chronic disease endpoints come from observational studies. This difference

BOX 3-1
Overview of Points Presented by Individual Speakers

- The current nutrient reference values (NRVs) process has generated considerable confusion because of its lack of transparency. Among other recommendations for future NRVs in Australia and New Zealand, a consultative group called for greater transparency in the decision-making process, including clear justification for the inclusion of experts on committees and clear documentation of the process of determining values (Clifton).
- Although risk assessment is at the heart of the Dietary Reference Intake (DRI) approach used in Canada and the United States, several key assumptions of this approach do not always fit for chronic disease endpoints (MacFarlane).
- As a first test of guiding principles laid out in the recently published report *Guiding Principles for Developing Dietary Reference Intakes Based on Chronic Disease* (NASEM, 2017a), a National Academies review of chronic disease endpoints in DRIs for sodium and potassium is already under way (King).

in the nature of the evidence that is available in the scientific literature is "not good or bad," MacFarlane said, "it just is what it is."

Continuing the focus on chronic disease endpoints, King highlighted major findings from a recently published National Academies of Sciences, Engineering, and Medicine report, *Guiding Principles for Developing Dietary Reference Intakes Based on Chronic Disease* (NASEM, 2017a). A major difference between traditional versus chronic disease DRIs, she pointed out, is that the latter are not warranted unless sufficient evidence exists, in contrast to traditional DRIs, which affect everyone. Recommendations in the National Academies report (2017a) covered how to select and judge chronic disease evidence (e.g., how to extrapolate intake–response data from one population to another); how chronic disease DRIs should be structured (e.g., as ranges, rather than single numbers); and the DRI process itself (e.g., continue to use the current DRI process, but, as a first step, conduct a thorough evidence-based systematic review of the nutrient and associated chronic disease risk). King remarked that, as a first test of these guiding principles, a National Academies review of chronic disease endpoints in DRIs for sodium and potassium was already under way.

FRAMEWORK CONSULTATION PROCESS: KEY ISSUES AND CONCLUSIONS[1]

Peter Clifton entered this field through his involvement with two consultations of the NRV framework in Australia, which itself was the end result of the 2005–2006 NRV review process.[2] The NRV framework adopted IOM recommendations almost completely, with what Clifton described as a whole array of new concepts being introduced. These included the estimated average requirement (EAR), the reference daily intake (RDI), and the adequate intake (AI), as well as acceptable macronutrient distribution range (AMDR). The introduction of AMDR in particular caused a lot of controversy and, according to Clifton, has not been used. Additionally, upper limits (ULs) were introduced for all nutrients and all age groups, again mostly as per the IOM recommendations. The introduction of the ULs caused controversy as well, he recalled, particularly with the regulatory agencies, as many of the limits were perceived to be set relatively arbitrarily and relatively low. But the major problem with the 2005–2006 NRV process, Clifton emphasized, was lack of transparency. Many people who contributed ideas about what the NRVs should be received no feedback, the reasons the 2005–2007 NRV review committee chose particular values were never recorded, and details about the process provided on the website were very limited. Clifton went on to describe these and other problems in more detail, actions taken since the consultations, and challenges with folate and vitamin D in particular.

Consultations and Recommendations

A main question addressed in the first consultation that Clifton was involved with (i.e., three public meetings in 2011 with targeted invitees from across Australia and New Zealand) was whether all of the NRVs should be reviewed or if only some of them should be reviewed and, if the latter, how the reviews should occur. The consultants found that stakeholders[3] felt there would be more opportunity for more detailed investigations and more substantive values (i.e., there would be more confidence in the values) if only a couple of nutrients were selectively reviewed.

---

[1] This section summarizes information presented by Peter Clifton, Ph.D., professor of nutrition, University of South Australia, Adelaide, Australia.

[2] The 2005–2006 NRV review process led to publication of *Nutrient Reference Values for Australia and New Zealand* in 2006. A PDF of that publication, plus updates since then, are available on the Australian Government's National Health and Medical Research Council website at https://www.nhmrc.gov.au/guidelines-publications/n35-n36-n37 (accessed December 14, 2017).

[3] Both here and in the Chapter 4 summary of Clifton's second presentation, "stakeholder" refers to the individuals consulted, as per the descriptions of the consultations in Australian Department of Public Health (2015).

Additionally, Clifton continued, stakeholders wanted more details on the NRV process, including how evidence is assessed, and more information on the purpose and use of NRVs.

Stakeholders also expressed ongoing confusion about inadequacy assessments of both individual and group intakes, including which particular NRV should be used and how it should be interpreted. For example, what is an acceptable level of intake below the EAR? Is 10 percent acceptable (i.e., 10 percent of the population with intakes below the EAR)? Clifton explained that, because people's dietary intakes are diverse, there will always be a percentage of the population below the EAR.

In addition to detailed descriptions of the EAR, stakeholders wanted detailed descriptions of the RDI and AI, and a detailed handbook on how to establish an EAR.

While stakeholders felt that the terminology that had been changed in 2005–2006 should not be changed again, as they had become accustomed to and had accepted that change, they felt that there were errors in scaling and extrapolation across the various age groups that needed to be corrected and that there needed to be more consistency in the application of scaling (i.e., across nutrients).

As Clifton had previously alluded, stakeholders also reported that the ULs caused problems with Food Standards Australia New Zealand, Australia's food regulatory agency, and that the ULs needed to be justified, not just borrowed from the IOM recommendations.

Finally, stakeholders requested a framework to guide expert working groups in how they should approach NRVs in the future. Clifton said that he had envisioned a limited handbook, but the framework ended up being a very detailed 80-page document (Australian Government Department of Health, 2015).

Following this first consultation, a series of recommendations were issued in 2012. The first was that there should be an immediate review of the chronic disease and macronutrient section of the 2006 NRVs. Many of the people who had been consulted felt there were many wrong statements in this section and that it needed more rigor. This review has not happened yet, Clifton noted. It was recommended that less comprehensive reviews be conducted for several nutrients as funding and time permit, namely B12, choline and pyridoxine, zinc, fluoride ULs, selenium ULs, energy, protein, and chloride. Additionally, it was recommended that a steering committee be established to oversee the review process and to act as an expert reference or advisory group and that a technical working group or consultant be engaged to develop a methodological framework.

In the second consultation, in 2012, again, Clifton emphasized, a major request on the part of those interviewed was greater transparency in the decision-making process. Stakeholders wanted clear justification for inclusion of experts on a committee, details for accepting or rejecting certain evidence, and clear documentation of all decisions and assumptions. Additionally, there was a call for development of robust methodologies to construct recommendations, particularly for nutrients with gaps in the data for specific population groups. It was suggested that in cases where there is a gap in the data, rather than doing a "guesstimate" and coming up with something not very robust, it should be communicated that no data are available and that a recommendation cannot be made.

Methodological Framework for the Review of Nutrient Reference Values

Realizing the need for a methodological framework to guide future reviews of NRVs, a committee was formed to develop this framework,[4] Clifton continued. The framework committee recommended that the first step of any NRV review should be to justify why that particular nutrient was chosen for review and what the issues are around it. For example, is there new evidence? Or are there new politics or policies (e.g., fortification) that justify a review? Then, after clearly defining the question, expert working groups need to identify which particular NRV(s) will be examined (e.g., UL, EAR), which age group will be considered (e.g., infants, children, adults), and whether the focus of the review will be nutritional deficiency or chronic disease prevention. Regarding the latter, Clifton remarked that the people consulted certainly wanted a chronic disease prevention component included in the NRV process, but separate from nutrition deficiency diseases. Additionally, the framework committee recommended the following:

- Clearly define and justify endpoints relevant for the assessment of nutrient deficiency and chronic disease prevention in advance of gathering the evidence.
- Derive recommendations for prevention of nutrient deficiency diseases using either the factorial or dose–response approach.
- Derive recommendations for chronic disease prevention using whatever evidence is available, including from both observational and intervention studies.
- Incorporate as much data as possible into meta-analyses or meta-regressions.

Clifton described the toxicologist on the framework committee as someone who was very strongly interested in harmful effects and who thought that the ULs that had been set during the 2005–2006 NRV pro-

[4] The framework is described in Australian Government Department of Health (2015).

cess were very arbitrary and had implied precision where precision did not really exist. Thus, the committee suggested a UL only where there is good evidence of an adverse effect. Otherwise, a "provisional UL" should be assigned where there is probably an adverse effect, but it is unclear what the value of the UL should be, or a "not determined" or "not required" UL should be assigned when there is no evidence of hazard or it is very unlikely that a hazard could occur. The latter designations are quite different from the current IOM model, Clifton remarked, and have not been adopted yet for any of the nutrients under review.

Lack of Harmonization Within Countries: Folate as an Example

Clifton explained that his interest in harmonization included harmonization within countries, not just among different expert working groups looking at the same nutrient. He cited folate as a good example of a nutrient whose recommended intakes have varied not only among countries, but within countries over time.

In Australia, the recommended intake was 330 micrograms (μg) free folic acid per day (for men and women) in 1977. Then it went up to 400 μg in 1980, then down to 200 μg of dietary folate equivalents (DFEs) in 1991. That was a very dramatic reduction, Clifton said, as 200 μg of DFE is essentially 100 μg of free folic acid. Then, in 1998, it went back up to 400 μg DFE. These changes occurred even though the criterion being used was the same, which was a red blood cell (RBC) folate level greater than 305 nanomoles per liter (nm/L). Similar changes have occurred over time in the United States, with the recommended level being reduced from 400 μg DFE in 1980 to 180 μg DFE in 1989. Again, Clifton said, this was a very dramatic reduction. The recommendation for pregnancy was reduced as well, from 800 μg DFE in 1980 to 400 μg DFE in 1989. Then, in 1998, the IOM recommended dietary allowance went back up to 400 μg DFE, as it did in Australia. The United Kingdom (UK) reference nutrient intake, however, has been set at 200 μg and the European Food Safety Authority population reference intake for folate at 330 μg.

Clifton reiterated that all of these values rely on the same biochemical indicator. Thus, it was not that the criteria differed that led to the variation in values, rather that the data were interpreted in what he described as "an un-harmonized kind of way."

Given these changes over time, Clifton raised the question: How should future expert working groups examine folate? How should they evaluate the data, apart from looking at all of it, especially given that data on deficiencies are very limited? Food folate is hard to measure, so there is really not even any accurate estimate of intake. That said, Clifton noted, it appears that the intake in Australia might be between 600 and 800 μg/day, which is well above the RDI. And folate assays of serum, particularly RBC folate, provide mixed results and, thus, their reliability is limited.

Because few EAR studies actually achieve a 50 percent adequacy level, rather than picking one or two of these studies and coming up with a guesstimate, Clifton suggested that many studies with different endpoints need to be integrated into a meta-regression to determine a best estimate. He was unaware of any meta-regression for folate. Added to the challenge is that the true coefficient of variation (CV) is unknown. The 10 percent CV that is being used is what he described as a "wild guesstimate" and may be far removed from actual reality. He suspected the actual CV might be a lot higher. Compared to the EAR, the RDI is a much simpler concept and may be an easier figure to derive, as it covers essentially the whole population.

Whether one should worry about folate in Western populations is difficult to know, Clifton opined. It is known that there is a folate-sensitive population with respect to neural tube defects, but that is a very small, select population. Discussing whether folate deficiency is common in the general population, Clifton mentioned a study of inpatients and outpatients at the Royal Prince Alfred Hospital in Sydney, Australia. Of 21,000 samples, 3.4 percent of the sampled population had low RBC folate levels (i.e., below 340 nmol/L). That sampling was conducted in April 2009, before folate fortification. After fortification, in 2010, the percentage of people with low RBC folate levels fell to 0.5 percent (0.16 percent in women of childbearing age). Thus, fortification changed the folate status of the population to virtually completely folate replete. Clifton concluded, "So it would appear that whatever the population are eating now is certainly adequate."

However, he continued, there is a bit of a mismatch between measured indicators of folate status versus intake indicators. Even with this virtually complete folate replete population, an estimated 10 percent of estimated intakes are below the EAR. "People are worried about this," he said.

In answer to his question, a future folate NRV expert working group will need to question all of the assumptions about how all of these figures were derived and check the data upon which the figures are based. A lot of the data are historical, he noted. Additionally, the difference between free folic acid found in supplements and the EAR/RDI DFEs is "totally unrecognized," he said. DFEs (i.e., food folate) are half as effective as folic acid or food fortified with folic acid.

In Clifton's opinion, the up-and-down nature of the folate recommendations over the years reflect either confusion about the endpoints or confusion about the data upon which the adequacy levels have been derived. Thus, regarding international harmonization of NRV folate review methodology, he emphasized the importance of agreement around which endpoints and which health markers to use, noting that there may be some new epigenetic markers of folate sufficiency. Other NRVs face similar issues. For example, recent changes in calcium and vitamin D recommendations similarly reflect a lack of clarity and confusion around appropriate endpoints.

Vitamin D

Vitamin D deficiency is epidemic across Australia, with millions of tests conducted yearly and millions of people being prescribed vitamin D. Thus, it is costing the country a large amount of money. Yet, Clifton remarked, it is very difficult to know whether this testing and prescribing is appropriate or inappropriate—whether it is of value or harm. In the United Kingdom, in 2016, a reference nutrient intake of 10 µg/day was established for all individuals above the age of 4 years. The aim, or endpoint, was to achieve a serum level for 25(OH)D of 25 nmol/L for 97.5 percent of the population, which Clifton said could be considered a very clear, firm, well-established endpoint. However, in Australia, using approximately the same endpoint of 27.5 nmol/L, the AI has been set at 5 µg/day for all individuals up to the age of 50 years, 10 µg/day for individuals between the ages of 50 and 70 years, and 15 µg for individuals over the age of 70 years. Thus, although the two countries use the same endpoint, they have issued different recommendations. He noted that it is difficult to know the extent to which either set of values takes into account sunshine synthesis of vitamin D. The U.S. values are different, with a recommendation of 15 µg/day for individuals up to the age of 70 years and 20 µg/day for individuals over the age of 70 years, but the endpoint is also different, such as a serum 25(OH)D level equal to or greater than 50 nmol/L.

In Clifton's opinion, vitamin D "would probably be the real challenge for harmonization," as it will require either persuading all countries to change their endpoints to align with the U.S. endpoint, probably in the absence of any evidence or in the presence of only a small amount of evidence, or persuading the National Academies to lower its intake recommendations.

ENDPOINTS: DIFFERENCES WHEN CONSIDERING DEFICIENCY VERSUS CHRONIC DISEASE[5]

In the 1990s, it was decided that Canada and the United States would move forward with a harmonized approach for setting nutrient reference values. The DRI framework was the basis of that approach, Amanda MacFarlane began. Prior to establishment of the DRI framework, both countries set their values independently, and their focus was on adequacy

[5] This section summarizes information presented by Amanda MacFarlane, Ph.D., research scientist, Health Canada, Ottawa, Ontario.

and prevention of deficiencies in the two populations. But with the DRI framework, there was an added focus, first, to ensure safe ULs of intake in addition to adequacy. These values were derived from data on apparently healthy populations, thus serving apparently healthy populations. However, in the 1980s, there was a growing recognition that nutrition has an effect on chronic disease. Thus, a second focus was added in the new framework: There should also be consideration of chronic disease risk reduction where sufficient data for efficacy and safety existed. This latter focus ended up posing more challenges than people had anticipated at the time, MacFarlane noted.

At the heart of the DRI framework is a risk-assessment approach. The first step, MacFarlane explained, is to demonstrate that there is a causal relationship between the intake of a particular nutrient and the endpoint of interest (e.g., disease of deficiency), then conduct a literature review and identify and select an indicator(s) of the endpoint that would be acceptable for setting a DRI. Once the causal relationship is determined, the next step is to establish the intake–response relationship, that is, find data showing that there are changes in the endpoint of interest as nutrient intakes increase. Once an intake–response model is established, then the DRI can be set. Other parts of the assessment include intake assessments of the population of interest and implications and special concerns for particularly susceptible or vulnerable populations. But the main part of the risk assessment, MacFarlane emphasized, is identifying the causal relationship and modeling the intake–response relationship.

There are a number assumptions inherent to this risk-assessment approach to setting DRIs, including

- the essentiality of the substance;
- evidence of causality and an intake–response relationship;
- that there is a threshold for adequacy and a threshold, or an assumed threshold, for adverse effects at the high end of intakes;
- that the relevant population is known;
- that there are biomarkers on the causal pathway between the intake of a particular nutrient and the disease of interest; and
- there is evidence that dictates the absolute nature of the risk for the disease of deficiency.

Between 1997 and 2005, DRI values generally were set to achieve adequate intakes and, when the data allowed, to prevent adverse effects from excessive intakes. But it was determined over and over again, MacFarlane recalled, that when these same assumptions were applied to a nutrient–chronic disease relationship, they did not always fit. "It was kind of like fitting a square peg into a round hole," she said. In the few cases where a nutrient–chronic disease relationship could be demonstrated, only an AI value was set. MacFarlane then went on to highlight in detail the limitations of several of these assumptions when applied to chronic disease endpoints.

Evidence of Causality: Deficiency Versus Chronic Disease Endpoints

Again, MacFarlane continued, one of the assumptions of the DRI approach is that there is a causal relationship between nutrient intake and an endpoint. When establishing causality or an intake–response relationship, normally the gold standard evidence is from an RCT and, ideally, from systematic reviews and meta-analyses of many RCTs (see Figure 3-1). Although establishing causality relies heavily on RCTs, it can be supported by evidence from intervention trials, metabolic/balance studies, and depletion/repletion studies, MacFarlane remarked. If these same study types are used to model an intake–response relationship as well, they need to include at least three doses. "I think it's fair to say," she said, "in terms of nutrition studies, a lot of this evidence is somewhat limiting. But this is what you need, and this is what was used primarily for setting [the 1997–2005] EAR values based on deficiency endpoints."

The challenge for chronic disease endpoints is that the nature of the

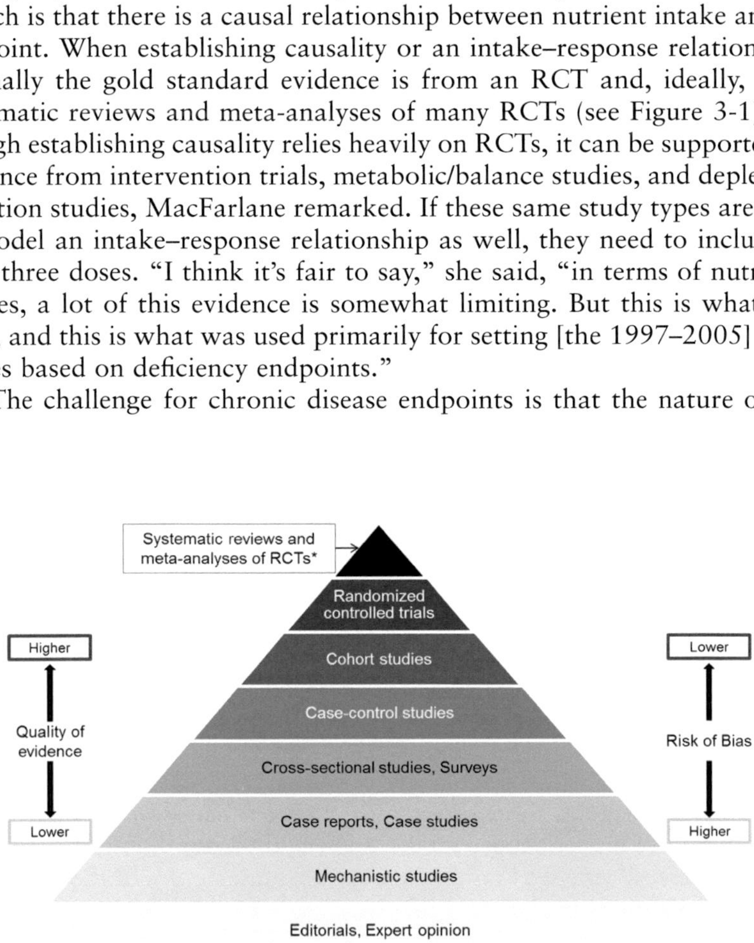

FIGURE 3-1 Evidence pyramid describing quality of evidence and risk of bias associated with different types of studies.
NOTES: RCT = randomized controlled trial; * Meta-analyses and systematic reviews of observational studies and mechanistic studies are also possible.
SOURCES: Presented by Amanda MacFarlane, HMD Workshop, Rome, Italy, September 21, 2017 (Yetley et al., 2016, by permission of Oxford University Press).

evidence available in the literature differs significantly. Most available evidence is associational, such as the cohort studies, case-control studies, and cross-sectional studies and surveys mentioned in Figure 3-1. "It's not bad or good. It just is what it is," MacFarlane said. The question, she said, is, "Can you establish a causal relationship or dose–response relationship in the absence of clinical trials?" Additionally, observational studies have a number of inherent biases and potential errors associated with each study type, such as confounding or selection bias and the limitations associated with self-reported intake data upon which these studies often rely.

Biomarkers on the Causal Pathway: Deficiency Versus Chronic Disease Endpoints

MacFarlane described that another assumption of the DRI framework is that there are biomarkers that are clearly on the causal pathway and that directly relate the intake status of a particular nutrient to the endpoint or disease of interest. She explained that examples of biomarkers on the clinical pathway include serum folate, serum 25(OH)D (vitamin D status), and serum ferritin. Having these biomarkers ensures a higher level of certainty when establishing a causal relationship between the intake of a particular nutrient and a disease. Ideally, MacFarlane added, the clinical outcome itself is directly observable, which is often the case with diseases of deficiency. Having this, plus an indicator of exposure directly related to that endpoint, makes it much more straightforward to demonstrate causality.

But, she said, when considering chronic disease risk, the situation is more complicated. First, chronic diseases have long pathological processes, making it difficult to demonstrate that an exposure is related to a particular clinical outcome. Additionally, sometimes a validated surrogate outcome has to be used instead of an actual clinical outcome as a predictor of the clinical outcome. There are also a number of nonvalidated intermediate outcomes that are possible predictors of the clinical outcome, but they have an even higher level of uncertainty. Either way, MacFarlane said, when the clinical outcome cannot be measured and, instead, one has to rely on either a surrogate or nonvalidated intermediate outcome, there is a higher level of uncertainty around the relationship between nutrient intake and chronic disease. A further issue is that currently there are very few validated surrogate outcomes, MacFarlane noted.

Data Available for Estimating Intake–Response Relationships: Deficiency Versus Chronic Disease Endpoints

Another assumption of the DRI framework is that there are absolute risks that affect all persons and all life-stage groups such that, as intake

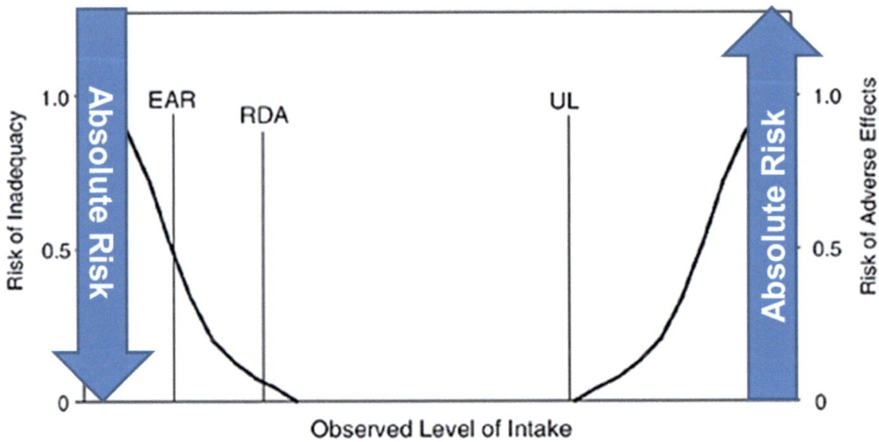

FIGURE 3-2 Risk of inadequacy (left y-axis) and risk of adverse effects (right y-axis) as a function of observed level of nutrient intake.
NOTE: EAR = estimated average requirement; RDA = recommended daily allowance; UL = upper limit.
SOURCES: Presented by Amanda MacFarlane, HMD Workshop, Rome, Italy, September 21, 2017. From IOM, 1994.

levels increase, the absolute risk of deficiency decreases (see Figure 3-2). Additionally, as also shown in Figure 3-2, there is an inflection point above which intake is associated with an increasing risk for an adverse effect. Thus, MacFarlane explained, depending on intake level, one can assume that there is a zero up to 100 percent risk of deficiency or adverse effects. She used an example from the 2011 vitamin D DRI report to illustrate. For all persons and all life stages (i.e., both younger and older age groups), as serum 25(OH)D levels (a biomarker of vitamin D status) increase, the risk of vitamin D deficiency bone problems decreases (IOM, 2011a).

However, this assumption does not apply when considering chronic disease risk. Not all persons are at risk of a chronic disease and not all life-stage groups are equally at risk of a chronic disease, MacFarlane explained. For example, the prevalence of diagnosed diabetes in Canada varies with age. Among the younger age groups, it is almost zero, and then it increases as age increases but only to a maximum prevalence of about 25 percent. In fact, often, less than 50 percent of a population is affected by any given chronic disease. So, again, an assumption of the DRI framework, in this case that every person of every life stage is affected by the same risk, does not apply when considering chronic disease.

Another difference with chronic disease risk, she added, is that it is often defined as relative risk, rather than absolute risk. In other words, there is no one who is at either zero or 100 percent risk. People are at either higher or lower risk compared to a baseline, or background, disease risk (Yetley et al., 2016). In the literature, changes in relative risk with changes in intake are often 10–20 percent, MacFarlane noted.

Thresholds for Adequacy and Upper Intake: Deficiency Versus Chronic Disease Endpoints

Yet another assumption that applies to deficiency endpoints is that there is an inflection point between inadequate and adequate intake levels. Yet, nutrient–chronic disease relationships often do not have inflection points. The relationship is often linear, with the greatest effect (i.e., change in risk) occurring at the tail(s) of the intake distribution (i.e., highest and/or lowest intakes have the largest effect). As an example, she described the association between fiber intake and coronary heart disease, where the relative risk of coronary heart disease decreases with increasing fiber intake (Threapleton et al., 2013). "If it lacks an inflection point," MacFarlane asked, "where are you supposed to set that EAR value?"

Similarly, it is assumed that there is a threshold for upper intake as well. But again, that is not always the case with a relationship between a particular nutrient and a chronic disease endpoint. For example, with saturated fat and low-density lipoprotein (LDL) cholesterol, as intake increases, LDL cholesterol increases linearly (IOM, 2002).

Interval Between Beneficial and Harmful Intakes: Deficiency Versus Chronic Disease Endpoints

The last assumption that MacFarlane described was that there is an interval between beneficial and harmful intakes. Again, like the other assumptions, this is not always the case with the relationship between intakes of a particular nutrient and a chronic disease. For example, the relationship between sodium and blood pressure is, again, an apparent linear relationship, with blood pressure continuing to increase as intake increases (IOM, 2005). "So where do you set a UL for a nutrient like this?" MacFarlane asked. At the time an AI for sodium was set (1.5 grams/day), it was based on adequacy for other nutrients and sweat losses, and the UL (2.3 grams/day) was based on the next higher dose in trials. MacFarlane said, "So, again, they did what they could with the data they had, but the chronic disease endpoints really challenged the DRI framework."

Additionally, because a single nutrient or single food substance potentially can be related to more than one chronic disease, there is also the potential for overlap of benefit and harm when considering the relationship between intake and the risk of more than one chronic disease. This is because the risk relationships between the nutrient and the different diseases could be different (Yetley et al., 2016). For example, each of the three theoretical chronic diseases (A, B, and C) illustrated in Figure 3-3 have different background risks. With increasing intake, the risks of disease A and disease C decrease, but the risk of disease B increases. "So what do you do with this kind of information?" MacFarlane asked. "Where would you set a DRI value for this kind of nutrient?"

Synopsis of the DRI Framework Approach

The DRI approach works well for estimating adequate intakes and adverse effects for essential nutrients, but it has been more challenging when using chronic disease endpoints, MacFarlane recapped. Chronic diseases are complex and can be influenced by many factors other than nutrients, including other food substances. Additionally, the available evidence relating nutrient intakes with a chronic disease can differ significantly from the

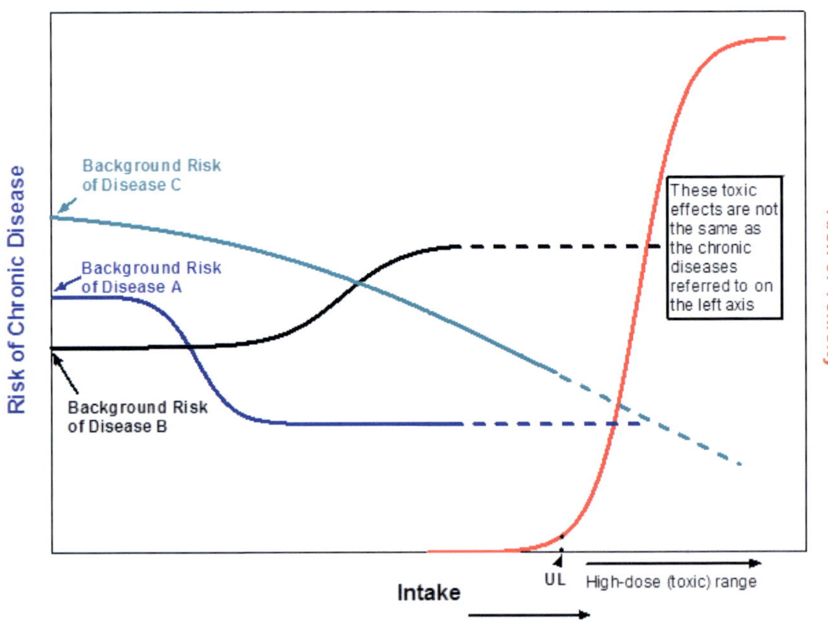

FIGURE 3-3 Differences in the risks of chronic diseases (left y-axis) versus toxicity (right y-axis) with increasing nutrient intake levels (x-axis).
SOURCES: Presented by Amanda MacFarlane and Janet King, HMD Workshop, Rome, Italy, September 21, 2017 (Yetley et al., 2016, by permission of Oxford University Press).

evidence that is available for establishing essentiality or toxicity of a given nutrient.

GUIDING PRINCIPLES FOR DEVELOPING DIETARY REFERENCE INTAKES BASED ON CHRONIC DISEASE: HIGHLIGHTS OF THE CONSENSUS REPORT[6]

A National Academies consensus report was published in August 2017 titled *Guiding Principles for Developing Dietary Reference Intakes Based on Chronic Disease* (NASEM, 2017a). The paradigm that the workshop planning committee used for their work was based on the "Options Report" (Yetley et al., 2016) and was similar to the paradigm the workshop planning committee was asked to follow, Janet King began. She noted that both she and Patrick Stover served on both the 2017 National Academies committee and the Options Report committee, thus ensuring that the historical development of concepts was not lost. King provided an overview of the 2017 National Academies committee's conversion of the concepts in Yetley et al. (2016) into guiding principles for how to develop DRIs for chronic disease.

The "Options Report": Differences Between Traditional DRIs and DRIs for Chronic Disease

The charge of the Options Report committee was to address options for dealing with the challenges encountered when establishing DRIs for chronic disease endpoints and to provide future guidance to DRI committees for judging nutrients and other food substances and chronic disease risk.

The first thing the committee had to do, King recalled, was think about how DRIs for the traditional nutrient recommendations differ from DRIs for chronic disease. The committee determined that a major difference is that traditional DRIs are for essential nutrients that are needed to prevent deficiencies. In other words, traditional DRIs affect everyone. If an individual's intake is inadequate, that individual will develop a nutrient deficiency. Because nutrient deficiencies are caused by single missing nutrients, they can be prevented through nutritional intervention, that is, by providing the missing nutrient. Chronic disease DRIs, in contrast, are not warranted unless there is sufficient evidence. That is, because the risk of acquiring a chronic disease because of dietary factors varies from individual to individual, there needs to be strong evidence that the risk occurs in the population of concern. Because chronic diseases are related to many

[6] This section summarizes information presented by Janet King, Ph.D., senior scientist, Children's Hospital Oakland Research Institute, Oakland, California.

risk factors in addition to diet and nutrition, including both genetic and environmental factors, nutritional interventions will only partly ameliorate the risk. King said, "The two parallel sets of DRIs are quite different in terms of their concepts."

King used one of the same figures that MacFarlane used in her presentation (see Figure 3-3) to emphasize that the relationship between nutrient intake and the risk for a chronic disease differs depending on which nutrient and which chronic disease are being addressed. For example, there may be a slight decrease in risk as intake increases (e.g., disease C in Figure 3-3), or there may be a sharp decline in risk that then levels off as intake continues to increase (e.g., disease A in Figure 3-3), or the risk may increase as intake increases (e.g., disease B in Figure 3-3). "It's a complex situation," King said.

Selecting and Judging the Chronic Disease Evidence

The National Academies consensus committee made two sets of primary recommendations: (1) how to determine whether specific levels of nutrients and other food substances can ameliorate chronic disease risk; and (2) how to develop DRIs based on chronic disease outcomes (NASEM, 2017a).

In its deliberations, the committee first had to figure out how to select and judge the evidence for a relationship between nutrition and chronic disease, King explained. It concluded that this involves, first, identifying the presence of a chronic disease by using either an acceptable diagnostic criteria or a surrogate biomarker of the disease. For example, with diabetes, one can determine if an individual has diabetes either by measuring blood glucose and insulin levels in the individual or by determining the level of hemoglobin A1c, a surrogate marker for the risk of diabetes. "So there are different ways that these analyses can be carried out," King said.

Next, the level of confidence of the relationship between the nutrients and other food substances and the chronic disease needs to be determined. The committee made two recommendations:

1. Use the Grading of Recommendations Assessment, Development and Evaluation (GRADE) evidence review system for that analysis, which is the same system being used at the World Health Organization (WHO) for evaluating the relationship between nutrient intakes and chronic diseases; and
2. The level of confidence for making a recommendation for a nutrients and other food substances level that reduces the risk of chronic disease should be based on at least a moderate level of certainty based on the GRADE system evaluation of the data.

"I think that may be a rather rigorous criteria to reach," King said, given that most of what she has seen in the literature has a lower level of confidence. "As we go forward and try to apply these guiding principles," she said, "we may find that we need to go back and rethink some of them."

Additionally, outcome indicators of the intake–response relationship need to be selected. In its report, the committee recommended using a single outcome indicator on the causal pathway, rather than multiple indicators. Again, using diabetes as an example, King suggested using only the hemoglobin A1c biomarker, which is on the causal pathway, and not to also include levels of glucose or insulin.

Finally, King reported, regarding how to extrapolate the intake–response data, the committee decided that this can only be done when data are extrapolated to similar populations with similar risks for the chronic disease. These data cannot be extrapolated widely to the whole population.

Structuring Chronic Disease DRIs

According to King, in its 2017 report the consensus committee decided that a DRI for chronic disease risk should be a range, rather than a single number, because the risk for a chronic disease can be spread over a range of intakes.

Additionally, the committee decided that if an increased chronic disease risk occurs only above the traditional UL, then there is no need to develop a DRI for chronic disease, because avoiding intakes above the UL will avoid that risk for chronic disease. So the UL is the cut point, King said. "If you don't see a risk for any disease unless the intake exceeds the UL, you don't need to worry about setting a DRI for that chronic disease."

Finally, there needs to be explicit and transparent descriptions of the health risks and benefits, especially when the benefits and harms of different chronic diseases overlap. "That concept needs to be very clearly laid out so individuals know how to apply the chronic disease DRIs," she said.

Recommendations Regarding the Process

The committee recommended continuing to use the current DRI process. Interestingly, King said, when they first started this work, she thought most of the committee was expecting to have to set up a totally different process for developing dietary recommendations for chronic disease. But as they delved into their deliberations, they began to see more clearly how the process could be incorporated into the structure already in place for developing nutrient recommendations.

The first step, King explained, is for the Agency for Healthcare Research and Quality to commission a thorough systematic review of the causal relationship between a nutrient and chronic disease. After that systematic review has been completed, then a specific nutrient-focused DRI committee will be assembled to determine if the existing evidence is sufficient to support developing chronic disease DRIs along with the traditional adequacy and toxicity DRIs. It is now recognized, she noted, that there may be a need for additional committee members who are more familiar with the disease process than with nutrient metabolism. Or, it may be necessary to appoint a subcommittee of individuals to this parent committee that includes the expertise needed to evaluate the disease process and translate that into a dietary recommendation.

This process will be applied for the first time with sodium and potassium, King said. The two nutrients will be reviewed separately, King clarified, not together or as a ratio. She clarified further that the review will determine whether there should be chronic disease DRIs for sodium and potassium *along with* traditional nutrient recommendations.

The first step will be a systematic review to determine if there is a causal relationship between sodium and a chronic disease. Then, after the systematic review has been completed, a DRI committee will be appointed, possibly with the assistance of a subcommittee, to judge the evidence using the GRADE system and to determine if the relationship between sodium and a single chronic disease outcome is causal in populations similar to those described in the evidence review. The recommendation for chronic disease endpoints was that a DRI committee would establish an intake range, not a single number, where the sodium-related chronic disease risk is minimal. If the sodium-related chronic disease risk occurs only above the traditional sodium UL, then no chronic disease DRI will be set. This will be the first test to "see if these guiding principles that were developed can be applied effectively," King concluded.

DISCUSSION

Following King's presentation, she, Clifton, and MacFarlane participated in an open discussion with the audience, as summarized here.

Chronic Disease DRI: A Range, Rather Than a Single Number

Ann Prentice asked about the concept of a chronic disease DRI range, as opposed to a single number, and how it will be interpreted by policy makers in their guidelines for the public. King replied that it will be similar to what is already being done with the dietary guidelines, which are often over a range and are not nearly as precise as what is trying to be established with the traditional DRIs. In King's opinion, it is wise not to have specific numbers, because variation even within a population at risk is fairly significant. Indeed, this was one of the major reasons that the 2017 National Academies consensus committee recommended using a range approach, rather than relying on single numbers.

Body Mass Index Issues for Chronic Disease DRIs

Lindsay Allen asked how body mass index (BMI) will be handled when developing chronic disease DRIs. King emphasized that the focus of the chronic disease evaluations will be on specific indicators, and she doubted that BMI would be such an indicator. However, she said that BMI "will likely track with the indicators that we are going to be evaluating." For example, people with BMIs above the normal range likely will have elevated blood pressure or elevated levels of hemoglobin A1c. But the DRI range will not be corrected for BMI.

Chronic Disease DRIs: Existing Conditions

Mary L'Abbé asked about preexisting conditions and whether dose–response curves might be different for individuals with preexisting conditions (e.g., individuals with hypertension versus without). "How would the model handle that? Could it conceivably come up with two different answers?" she asked. King replied that she was hoping that the GRADE system will be able to eliminate a number of relationships that might exist, such as that one. "I thought we were being rigorous when we said we were going to use the GRADE system," she said, "and also when we said we wanted it to have at least a moderate level of certainty."

Why Hypertension?

Clifton asked why hypertension was chosen as the endpoint for the first chronic disease DRI review (i.e., for sodium and potassium), rather than a hard endpoint such as a heart attack or stroke. He opined that most people will accept that an increased intake will elevate your blood pressure. However, he pointed out, hypertension is just an intermediate health outcome, one that is affected by many different factors. "The real argument is," he said, "does that matter in terms of hard endpoints?"

"We recognize that, and we actually spent a fair amount of time thinking that through," King responded. The committee decided that using those clinical endpoints is not going to be very helpful in terms of setting up a relationship with nutrient intakes, so they recommended looking for a surrogate marker instead. Clifton pressed his point further: Surrogate markers may not relate to the hard endpoints. "That's the real crux of the question," he said. King agreed that this will be a challenge that DRI committees will need to deal with when they develop their surrogate markers.

Patrick Stover, who, along with King, also served on the 2017 National Academies committee, added that there was also a lot of discussion about what the right endpoints are and that, whenever possible, they should be "person-important" outcomes, that is, they should be clinically meaningful outcomes. It is when those are not available, he said, that "you have to start walking back."

MacFarlane clarified that chronic disease DRIs are different values than deficiency DRIs. So the traditional EAR and UL are maintained, with the chronic disease DRIs being in addition to those other values. Her understanding of the guiding principles was that if the data are not sufficient or not available then chronic disease values would not be set.

A Harmonized Framework for Low- and Middle-Income Countries

Catherine Leclercq asked if a framework was going to be developed for countries that will not be able to develop standards from primary data, that is, for low- and middle-income countries who will need to derive intake values from the United States, Canada, Australia, WHO, or elsewhere. King replied that chronic disease issues vary drastically from country to country, particularly when comparing low- and middle-income countries to higher-income countries. In her opinion, it has to be done within countries by experts in those countries who have the data and understand the data. MacFarlane added, "That's the beauty of the guiding principles." They are not specific values that are being set, rather principles that can be applied at a country or region level.

Evidence from Observational Studies Versus RCTs: Chronic Disease Endpoints

George Wells commented on the evidence pyramid that MacFarlane showed during her presentation (see Figure 3-1), with RCTs on top and observational studies in the lower tiers. He asked how much evidence would be taken from RCTs versus observational studies when dealing with chronic disease endpoints. MacFarlane reiterated her expectation that more evidence will be coming from observational studies than from RCTs, given how few nutrition RCTs relate to particular nutrients and chronic disease endpoints. The challenge comes from the complexity of the development of chronic diseases over not just years, but decades, and the difficulty in establishing an exposure relationship with those diseases. She suggested that future studies may need to focus on at-risk populations of individuals who have not yet developed clinical outcomes but who can be identified on the basis of validated surrogate endpoints.

The GRADE System

Wells commented on the number of different ways that GRADE can evaluate risk of bias or quality and asked if the 2017 National Academies committee had decided on the GRADE system input yet. King was not part of the 2017 National Academies GRADE subcommittee and was unable to answer the question, but she commented on the considerable analysis and detail addressed when deliberating about how GRADE should be set up, how it should be used, what endpoints should be considered, and other related factors.

Folate: Assessment of Indicators

Ruth Charrondiere expressed fascination with Clifton's data showing that among approximately 21,000 people (i.e., patients at the Royal Prince Alfred Hospital in Sydney) only 3 percent were folate deficient. She wondered if there were also any data showing what these same individuals' folate intakes were prior to hospitalization so their RBC folate levels measured at the hospital could be correlated with folate intake estimates. She suspected that more than 3 percent of the general Australian population would show up as folate deficient based on folate intake estimates.

Clifton replied that, while it was a different population, the average folate intake measured in a later survey was around 700 mg/day, which he said was "well and truly above the RDI." Even so, within that population, 10 percent were below the EAR. But that is to be expected in a population where young people do not consume fruits and vegetables. "That's the reality," he said. "It is quite possible to have a high intake and a certain percentage below the EAR, because of the nature of people's dietary intake." In his opinion, the Australian population is replete even without fortification. He clarified that fortification is not being done for folate sufficiency, rather it is a targeted intervention across the population to achieve a reduction in neural tube defects. It has, he said, "nothing to do with folate endpoints in red cells."

MacFarlane underscored the need to decide, when assessing indicators being used to set nutrient reference values (for any nutrient), what the gold standard is. For folate, the microbiological assay is "really the gold standard," she said. That was the method that WHO used to establish cutoffs for both deficiency and for prevention of neural tube defects. Hospitals usually use protein binding assays, which are very different. In the absence of conversion factors between estimates derived from a gold standard versus a regular platform, she urged serious consideration about whether data should be used or not.

**Reality Check:
Are Chronic Disease RDIs Achievable with Healthy Food Intake?**

Charrondiere also asked if there would be what she referred to as a "reality check" when chronic disease DRIs are set. That is, will there be an additional step to check to see that the DRIs are achievable with a healthy food intake? If the recommended levels can only be achieved through fortification, she said, "there might be something wrong in our whole methodology."

Clifton responded that, at least with folate, the normal diet in Australia is quite adequate. He reiterated that fortification was done for a totally different purpose, not for normalization of the diet per se. MacFarlane added that in Canada, in the 1970s, which was the last time a biomarker analysis of folate was conducted, about 25 percent of the population was demonstrating deficiency. With fortification, now there is less than 1 percent deficiency. More generally, she agreed that a reality check is important, but suggested that the DRIs already do that to a degree. Usually when an EAR is set, an intake assessment of the population is conducted to see where the population is. When the values are different than what intakes indicate, she suspected that some of the difference relates to what she called "that disconnect between intake and status biomarkers." She suggested, "Perhaps we need more research to establish what those true relationships are between intake and actual status."

4

Current Models for Establishing Intake Recommendations

OVERVIEW

In addition to the presentations summarized in Chapter 3, session 1 included a panel discussion, "Current Models for Establishing Intake Recommendations." The panel was moderated by Hasan Hutchinson. Hutchinson and three other panelists from different regions of the world described their experiences with the harmonization of approaches to establishing nutrient intake recommendations. This chapter summarizes their presentations and the discussion that followed, with major points highlighted here and in Box 4-1.

Hutchinson provided an overview of the joint Canadian–U.S. effort to develop harmonized Dietary Reference Intakes (DRIs), an effort that began in 1994 and which continues to this day. By 2005, he said, a fairly complete set of DRIs had been established, but with no formal process to keep the DRIs up to date. Thus, a joint steering committee developed a structured process for deciding which nutrients to update based on changes in evidence, new methodologies, and other criteria. As King had previously discussed (summarized in the previous chapter), the sodium and potassium DRI reviews will be updated first, using the new guiding principles for chronic disease endpoints.

Clifton summarized recommendations issued in 2012 for South Australia and New Zealand, actions taken since then, and challenges faced. The 2012 recommendations included an immediate review of the chronic disease and macronutrient section, less comprehensive reviews of some micronutrients (e.g., the upper limit [UL] for fluoride), and greater transparency in the decision-making process. Among other actions taken since then, a fluoride

BOX 4-1
Overview of Points Presented by Individual Speakers

- The joint Canadian–U.S. effort to develop harmonized Dietary Reference Intakes (DRIs) began in 1994 and continues to this day but with a new structured process for deciding which nutrients to update based on changes in evidence, new methodologies, and other criteria (Hutchinson).
- Among other actions taken since recommendations were issued for future nutrient reference values in Australia and New Zealand, a fluoride working group was established, and its work is clearly documented and available online. The work was a 2-year process and illustrates the time-consuming nature of a review of a relatively targeted area, but one done comprehensively (Clifton).
- Among other changes that South Korea has made with its DRIs over the years, since the first set was issued in 1962, the 2015 committee has used Korean-specific data from the literature. For international harmonization, core processes and methods can be standardized but should be adaptable to country-specific data (Paik).
- Although the United Kingdom Scientific Advisory Committee on Nutrition generally derives its recommendations using the same basic estimated average requirement framework that other countries use, the recent vitamin D recommendation required setting a new "population protective value." One of the greatest challenges in this work is the acceptance, interpretation, and understanding of new technology (Prentice).

working group was established. Its work, all of which Clifton said is clearly documented and available online, was approved in 2016 by the Australian National Health and Medical Research Council. The fluoride work took almost 2 years, illustrating for Clifton the time-consuming nature of a review of a relatively targeted area, but one done comprehensively.

Next, Hee Young Paik described how recommended dietary allowances (RDAs) in South Korea have changed over the past several decades, beginning in 1962 when the first RDAs were published. Most recently, in 2015, a committee comprising 78 members, with subcommittees for different nutrients, reviewed the DRIs for 36 nutrients. In 2005, members of the Korean Nutrition Society decided that it was time to change the concept from RDAs to DRIs. Paik emphasized the 2015 committee's use of Korean-specific data from the literature. For international harmonization, she suggested that core processes and methods be standardized by having an international expert group review the international literature, but be adaptable to specific countries, such as by having an expert group in each country review local literature using a standardized methodology.

Finally, Ann Prentice described past and current nutrition risk assessment work by the United Kingdom (UK) Scientific Advisory Committee on Nutrition. She emphasized the committee's focus is on risk assessment, not risk management. The committee's dietary recommendations are derived using the same basic estimated average requirement (EAR) framework that other speakers have been describing, according to Prentice, and have been since 1981, when the United Kingdom's first reference nutrition intakes (RNIs) were published. The committee's recent vitamin D recommendation, however, went beyond the traditional EAR and RNI framework, because of the risk of bone health problems below a particular intake value and the desire for everyone in the population to reach that value year-round and not just when sun exposure is greatest. Instead, they set a "population protective value." In her experience, Prentice has found that one of the biggest problems is the acceptance, interpretation, and understanding of new terminology.

DIETARY REFERENCE INTAKES: HARMONIZED NUTRIENT STANDARDS FOR CANADA AND THE UNITED STATES[1]

The Canadian–U.S. joint effort to develop DRIs began in 1994. The rationale for a common set of values, Hasan Hutchinson explained, included the expanded base of specialized scientific expertise made available through collaboration; that the science underlying nutrient requirements knows no borders; and that the two populations have similar dietary needs. Additionally, it made sense to develop similar approaches to help with trade-related matters around nutrition

According to Hutchinson, since 1994, even though the two countries have separate DRI steering committees, all of the decisions to commission DRI reviews have been made jointly, with a series of six nutrient-focused reports released between 1997 and 2005. DRIs were developed for all macronutrients as well as 35 vitamins and minerals. In 2011, updated DRIs for calcium and vitamin D were released.

Structured Process for Updating DRIs

In 2012, a decision was made with input from both steering committees to develop a structured process for deciding which nutrients needed to have updated DRIs. Rather than conducting a comprehensive review of all the nutrients one by one, it was decided to develop an open nomination process to identify priority nutrients to update. Hutchinson explained

[1] This section summarizes information presented by Hasan Hutchinson, Ph.D., N.D., director general, Office of Nutrition Policy and Promotion, Health Canada, Ottawa, Ontario.

that nominations can be received from inside or outside of the government and need to include a rationale indicating where there has been a change of evidence, a need for updating because of policy implications, a change in methodology, or some other reason to reexamine a DRI. The Canadian and American committees then examine the nominations to see if they meet a set of nomination criteria. Together, the committees prioritize nutrients for further consideration and form working groups to conduct an in-depth assessment for each candidate nutrient. Each working group includes U.S. and Canadian experts. Following in-depth assessments, joint Canadian–U.S. decisions are made regarding which candidate nutrients should be considered for further assessment. If the decision is made to update a particular nutrient, the Agency for Healthcare Research and Quality is tasked to conduct a systematic review. With sufficient evidence from the systematic review, the National Academies would then be contracted to conduct a DRI review.

Canada and the United States decide separately how the information is to be applied in their respective countries. The hope, Hutchinson said, is that the recommendations in these reports can be directly applied to dietary guidance. He added they are also used to make other decisions, such as decisions about fortification and supplementation.

Hutchinson remarked that while the 2013 nomination process received 26 nominations for a total of 16 nutrients, which resulted in a short list of nutrients to move forward, the steering committees identified a need to address the challenge of chronic disease endpoints. This led to the development of guiding principles for developing DRIs based on chronic disease endpoints (NASEM, 2017a). Hutchinson referred to the earlier presentations by MacFarlane and King (summarized in Chapter 3), noting, as they had, that the sodium/potassium DRI review, initiated in the fall of 2017, is the first to use these new guiding principles.

SOUTH AUSTRALIA AND NEW ZEALAND[2]

In 2012, several recommendations were put forward regarding the nutrient reference value (NRV) process in Australia and New Zealand. The first, Peter Clifton began,[3] was that an immediate review should be conducted of the chronic disease and macronutrient section. The Departments of Health in Australia and New Zealand did not do this, Clifton said. A second recommendation was that a less comprehensive review should be

[2] This section summarizes information presented by Peter Clifton, Ph.D., professor of nutrition, University of South Australia, Adelaide, South Australia, Australia.

[3] For additional details on these recommendations and the consultative process that led to them, see the Chapter 3 summary of Clifton's earlier presentation.

conducted for B12, choline and pyridoxine, zinc (after findings are released from the International Zinc Nutrition Consultative Group [IZiNCG]),[4] the tolerable upper intake level (UL) for fluoride and selenium, energy, protein, and chloride, as funding and time permit. Third, it was recommended that there be greater transparency in the decision-making process, including clear justification for inclusion of experts and determination of nutrient values. And finally, it was recommended that there be clear documentation of all underlying decisions, evidence, assumptions, and rounding processes.

An advisory committee was set up by a steering committee from the Departments of Health in Australia and New Zealand to decide on the priority nutrients. But they provided no justification for why they chose the nutrients they did, Clifton stated. A fluoride expert working group was set up to focus on both the UL and adequate intake (AI) for fluoride, which had been recommended. However, a sodium expert working group was also set up, which had not been recommended. It was communicated only indirectly that the reason for setting up the sodium expert working group was to model chronic disease methodology, which Clifton noted is also what Health Canada and the National Academies are currently doing. That review is still in progress. It has been 2 years, so "it's obviously quite a thorny area," Clifton said.

In addition to the fluoride and sodium expert working groups, an iodine expert working group was also set up. As with sodium, iodine was not on the recommended list of priority nutrients. And again, there was no published reason for the choice other than the fact that, with fortification, it is a reasonable decision to review required levels. However, in Clifton's opinion, that decision also possibly reflects steering committee members' interest in iodine.

Finally, although there was some suggestion that carbohydrates be reviewed, there was no interest among potential expert working group members to move that review forward. Carbohydrates are viewed as a difficult and thorny area, a view that Clifton said he shared. Nonetheless, he suspected that similar lack of interest will likely be an issue for other macronutrients, as well as micronutrients, in the future.

The fluoride working group followed the recommendations of the new framework beautifully,[5] Clifton continued. They performed a systematic review to obtain all available evidence; they were provided administrative support and research assistants; all of their actions were clearly documented

[4] Details about IZiNCG, an international group focused on reducing global zinc deficiency, are provided at http://www.izincg.org (accessed April 25, 2018).

[5] See the summary of Clifton's earlier presentation in Chapter 3 for additional details about the new framework (Australian Government Department of Health, 2015) and the consultative process that led to its development.

and available online; the public consultation and comments are available online; and the paper was reviewed by methodological experts, as well as by experts in fluoride, dentistry, and pediatric health. The National Health and Medical Research Council approved the report in March 2017. The entire process took about 2 years. Even though the focus of the work was a relatively targeted area (i.e., AI and UL for fluoride for children between 2 and 8 years of age), the review was very comprehensive. "Clearly it's a time-consuming exercise," Clifton said.

It remains to be seen what will happen with the sodium review and what other additional reviews will be chosen in the future, he concluded. He expressed disappointment that the funders did not follow the input provided by expert consultants.

SOUTH KOREA: 2015 DIETARY REFERENCE INTAKES FOR KOREANS[6]

The first Korean recommended dietary allowances (KRDAs) were published in 1962 by the Korean Regional Office of the United Nations' Food and Agriculture Organization (FAO), Hee Young Paik said as she began her history of nutrient standards in Korea. That same office issued two subsequent revisions. Later, the Korea Institute for Health and Social Affairs, a government institute, published the fourth and fifth editions in 1985 and 1989, respectively. Then, the Korean Nutrition Society (KNS) took over responsibility, publishing the next two editions in 1995 and 2000. When preparing for the 2005 KRDAs, Paik said, members of the society felt it was time to change from RDAs to DRIs. The first DRI committee (i.e., the 2005 committee), of which Paik served as chair, reported values for 34 nutrients. The 2010 committee reported on 35 nutrients. Paik remarked that although it had been an unwritten rule of the KNS that the RDA and DRIs would be revised every 5 years, the 2010 National Nutrition Management Act legally mandated the Ministry of Health and Welfare to publish revised Korean DRIs (KDRIs) every 5 years.

The 2015 Korean DRIs

The Ministry of Health and Welfare set up a committee known as the General Administration Committee, composed of government officials and representatives from the nutrition community, as well as other stakeholders, to publish the 2015 KDRIs. The General Administration Committee's job,

[6] This section summarizes information presented by Hee Young Paik, Sc.D., director, Center for Gendered Innovations in Science and Technology Research, Korea Federation of Women's Science and Technology Associations, Seoul, South Korea.

Paik explained, was mainly to ensure that the process was going well and to resolve any problems that arose. The KNS remained responsible for the actual scientific process of establishing the values (i.e., reviewing scientific evidence on nutrients, data on age and physical standards, and data on dietary intake). The KNS committee that conducted the evidence and data review (the 2015 KDRIs Establishment Committee) had several subcommittees, including 1 for age and physical standards, 1 for applications (e.g., food group guide), 8 for energy and macronutrients, 13 for vitamins, 14 for minerals, 1 for infants, and a review subcommittee. The total number of members was 78.

The 2015 KDRIs cover estimated energy requirements (EERs), acceptable macronutrient distribution ranges (AMDRs), and EARs, RNIs, AIs, and ULs for vitamins and minerals. The total number of nutrients covered was 36, which Paik noted was fewer than the number of U.S. and Canadian DRIs (40 in 1997–2011), but more than in most other countries (e.g., Japan had 31 in 2015, Germany/Switzerland/Austria had 27 in 2015, and Australia/New Zealand had 33 in 2005).

Changes between the 2010 and 2015 KDRIs, Paik noted, include that the upper range of the carbohydrate AMDR was lowered to 65 percent in the 2015 KDRIs, compared to 70 percent in the 2010 KDRIs, and the upper range of the total fat AMDR for adults 18 years and older was increased to 30 percent, compared to 25 percent in the 2010 KDRIs.

The strategy for setting the KDRIs is similar to the process developed by the United States and Canada, Paik continued, that is, it involves systematic evidence review of the international literature and meta-analyses when possible. Plus, it involves a rigorous review of the Korean literature, using the same level of judgment that is used for the international literature, and the use of Korean data, especially for body size and dietary intake data. While the processes are similar, Paik remarked that not all components of the DRI process used in the United States and Canada are applicable to the KDRIs. For example, while the methods and biological characteristics are adoptable, particular references to population and country characteristics are not.

Thoughts on International Harmonization

Paik concluded by offering some suggestions for international harmonization. Generally, she suggested that core processes and methods be standardized, but these should be able to be adapted by specific countries. For example, she suggested that international experts not only review the international literature and make their reviews available to each country, but also develop a standardized methodology for literature review. Expert groups in each country can then use this methodology to review local literature (i.e., literature published locally in their own language) and provide feedback to the international committee regarding their local literature review. This two-way sharing of literature reviews "will make our work more complete," Paik said. Additionally, she suggested that international experts provide guidance on standards for national resource data, such as guidelines for national surveys in nutrition, body size, and dietary practices. Local expert groups could also use guidelines on food composition tables and database methodology. Finally, she suggested periodic updating of DRIs.

UNITED KINGDOM[7]

Ann Prentice described the UK Scientific Advisory Committee on Nutrition, of which she was currently chair, as a committee of independent experts who are appointed and who are not employed by the government. In many ways, she said, they are accountable to the whole of the UK government, across a multitude of departments and agencies. Their focus is specifically in risk assessment in diet, nutrition, and health. Risk management, in contrast, is the role of government. Although the committee is sometimes invited to help government authorities understand information being communicated by the committee, it is the responsibility of those authorities, not the committee, to make a decision and consider how to implement their decision.

Nor is the committee involved with aspects related to adverse effects, Prentice clarified further, although there are joint working groups that collaborate on issues that overlap. As an example, she mentioned a recent sodium and potassium joint working group.

The committee's dietary recommendations are very much based on the framework that previous speakers had been discussing, as they have been since 1991 when the original set of RNIs were first developed, Prentice remarked. (An RNI is the amount of nutrient that is enough to ensure that the needs of 97.5 percent of a population are being met.) In addition to RNIs, the UK dietary reference values (DRVs) also include EARs and lower reference nutrient intakes (LRNIs; an LRNI is the amount of nutrient that is enough for a small percentage of people in a population who have low requirements). She noted that LRNIs are a useful monitoring tool for the UK National Diet and Nutrition Survey.

When evaluating and synthesizing the evidence, the committee is required to consider the entirety of the data, but it uses what Prentice

[7] This section summarizes information presented by Ann Prentice, OBE, Ph.D., DUS, director, Medical Research Council (UK) Elsie Widdowson Laboratory, University of Cambridge, England.

described as a formalized and transparent hierarchy framework. At the beginning of each work package, the committee is obliged to consider and decide exactly how they will move forward. Then, depending on the nutrient under consideration, the committee may decide, for example, to use only systematic reviews or to also include animal data. Often, the committee uses systematic reviews from Canada and the United States as a basis for its evaluation and then looks for additional, more recent data. It also examines the assumptions of the existing systematic reviews to determine whether they are appropriate for the particular piece of work the committee is addressing. As an example of its use of a different set of assumptions, in a recent review of weight loss and carbohydrates, the committee decided to consider only those studies with 12-month outcomes, not 3-month outcomes.

With its recent vitamin D review, the UK committee felt the need to go beyond the traditional RNI/EAR framework. Specifically, Prentice explained, based on the 25(OH)D vitamin D biomarker, the working group concluded that evidence indicated a risk of bone health problems below a particular level. Recognizing that most people would exceed that level, certainly in summer, the committee also recognized that there are ethnic minorities in the United Kingdom with no seasonal variation in 25(OH)D. To address the risk of bone health problems across the entire population, the committee set what it called a "population protective level" of 25(OH)D for the entire population to be above year-round. The committee used experimental intake–response data from studies commissioned by the UK government to develop this value. Its abandonment of the traditional framework in the case of vitamin D raises questions around terminology, particularly the acceptance of new terminology, that Prentice thought worth considering during this meeting.

In conclusion, Prentice mentioned that in addition to their recent vitamin D publication and forthcoming sodium/potassium publication, the committee is also currently working on saturated fat, folate, iodine, complementary infant feeding and cognitive development, and health in old age. Additionally, she expressed curiosity about how consideration of chronic disease endpoints will move forward and opined that although current DRVs are largely based on avoidance of deficiency, chronic disease is not a separate challenge. Finally, she emphasized, "I have found the biggest problem has been, in many ways, trying to interpret the terminology that we as nutrition scientists and nutritionists use to my clinical colleagues and, indeed, to my toxicological colleagues." She observed, in addition, how various agencies are hesitant to accept not just new terminology, but also new models.

DISCUSSION

Following the panel presentations, the panel was opened to discussion and questions from the audience, as summarized here.

New Terminology: Acceptance and Understanding

In response to Prentice's remarks about the acceptance of new terminology, Clifton commented that when there are huge differences in terminology among Europe, the United Kingdom, and the United States, it is difficult to know which terminology is the best one to accept. Most people choose to continue using what they have been using, he observed. However, if there is agreement on a specific terminology, he said, "Australia would certainly follow that."

Paik added that most people want very clear communication around dietary standards. When South Korea changed from RDA to DRI terminology, it took a lot of work to convince people, including nutritionists and dietitians, that the change was needed. An added challenge in non-English speaking countries, she pointed out, is the development of new words to accompany changed English terminology. But, she said, "I think we have to all realize that things evolve, our knowledge evolves, our thinking evolves." Communicating these changes is challenging, but necessary.

Change in UK Vitamin D Recommendation: Real-World Impact

Clifton wondered whether, since the United Kingdom's new vitamin D guidelines were published, recommending 10 micrograms per day across essentially the whole population, there has been any conspicuous change in food fortification. Or, have pharmacies noticed an increased uptake of vitamin D supplements? He said that he was asking, essentially, "Does what the scientists and the nutritional community advocate have any effect in the real world?"

Prentice replied that it has been too short a time to see whether there has been a change in intake. Those data will come from the United Kingdom's continuous National Diet and Nutrition Survey, and the most recent data are not available yet. However, she said, there has been a change in the way that government recommendations are being published. But there has been no change in thinking about vitamin D fortification, she added. She mentioned the folic acid recommendations that were made 20–25 years ago. Today, she said, "that one is still rumbling on. I'm afraid nothing happens."

Clifton commented on the very positive press coverage of the new vitamin D guidelines. He said, "You would think people reading that might think, 'I'd better go and get some vitamin D from the supermarket.'"

Prentice agreed that vitamin D will be more available in the United Kingdom than it has been in the past. In the past, it was available only through prescription. Now it can be bought off the shelf. However, she added, based on past UK survey data, it is what she referred to as the "worried well" who take supplements even though they do not need them, and the people who really need them who do not take them.

Hutchinson commented that, in Canada, based on 2015 data, they should know within the next year whether there have been any changes in vitamin D intake patterns. They are ready to move forward on fortification, he said, if necessary, but they want to have an idea of what the consumption patterns are before they make any changes.

The Value of a Regional Approach to Setting NIVs

John Muyonga pointed out that one of the benefits of harmonization for developing countries is the sharing of resources and the opportunity for regional, as opposed to national, nutrition intake values (NIVs). Currently, many countries are using FAO and the World Health Organization guidelines because they do not have the resources to put together national NIV committees. Referring to Paik's mention of the 78 members on the committee that developed the 2015 KNRVs, Muyonga said that some countries do not even have 78 nutrition experts.

Paik agreed that the development of some kind of regional cooperation would be very helpful, given that diets and nutrition-related health problems are often similar across a region. For example, when South Korea developed its first set of KDRIs in 2005, at that time Japan was similarly adopting the DRI terminology. The two countries did not share the output of their work, partly because the KDRI work was done by the Korean Nutrition Society, a nongovernmental organization of scientists, whereas Japan's DRIs were set up by the governmental National Institute of Nutrition and Health. However, she said, "We had some communication." When asked by Clifton whether there had been any collaboration with China, given all of the nutrition intake data being collected in China (e.g., the PURE Study), Paik replied that, at the time, China had not yet established DRIs. She predicted that, in the future, there would be some communication.

Additionally, acknowledging that she was unsure who would be responsible for running such resources, Paik suggested that each country contribute to an international research literature repository so the international community has at its disposal not just English literature, but local literature as well.

Hutchinson reiterated that, while Canada and the United States obviously take a bit of a regional approach, entering usual intake data from both countries into the report analyses, risk management is very much handled by the individual countries. "We can sometimes have different approaches using the same data," he said.

Anna Lartey observed that while it is the developed countries that are really working in this area, every country has its own national academy of science. She called for efforts to work with these national academies so each country can develop its own original nutrient intake recommendations and suggested that the U.S. National Academies could play a big role in this.

South Korean Change in Carbohydrate Recommendation

During her presentation, Paik had described how the upper range of the carbohydrate AMDR was lowered to 65 percent in the 2015 KDRIs, compared to 70 percent in the 2010 KDRIs. She also said the upper range of the lipid total fat AMDR for adults 18 years and older was increased to 30 percent, compared to 25 percent in the 2010 KDRIs. Muyonga asked why the carbohydrate and fat AMDRs were changed in the 2015 KDRIs. Paik replied that the former UL of 70 percent for carbohydrates was very high, given many recent reports of the associated risks for chronic disease. Plus, there has been a trend toward decreased carbohydrate consumption. In addition to lowering the UL of the recommended carbohydrate distribution, they also felt that it would be appropriate to modify the ratio of fat to carbohydrates for adults.

Models for Recommendations for Infants and Children

When asked by Inga Thorsdottir how the UK Scientific Advisory Committee on Nutrition established intake recommendations for infants and children, Prentice replied that because there is relatively little evidentiary data for children those recommendations are made generally by extrapolation and by weight. But many of the committee's recent deliberations have not even required that, she added. For example, while carbohydrates and their energy report certainly did, there is no evidence to suggest that there is any difference in the requirement for vitamin D. For Prentice, the question raised yet another question, one regarding physiological variance in general. There is so little information on variation in physiology, she lamented, with most available data being based on means.

Paik added that, in Korea, one of the 2015 KDRI subcommittees was for infants, because infants' diets differ than those of other age groups.

Developing Food-Based Dietary Guidelines

Rune Blomhoff remarked that different food-based dietary guidelines (e.g., those developed by the American Institute for Cancer Research or the World Cancer Research Fund) are developed using different methodologies. He asked how nutrient recommendations can be integrated with these different food-based dietary guidelines. Hildegard Przyrembel agreed that NRVs are a prerequisite to food-based dietary guidelines. She referred to a 2006 FAO paper and European Food Safety Authority (EFSA) opinion piece on the principles of formulating food-based dietary guidelines. The EFSA scientific opinion, she noted, provides a stepwise approach. She emphasized, however, "You cannot globalize it." It can only be done on a national basis. Hutchinson added that many countries are in fact following the FAO model, which, he explained, incorporates the EFSA stepwise approach, for developing food-based dietary guidelines.

5

Exploring Approaches to Evaluating the Evidence

OVERVIEW

The focus of session 2, moderated by Ann Prentice, was on approaches to evaluating evidence in the scientific literature. This chapter summarizes the session 2 presentations and discussion, with major points highlighted here and in Box 5-1.

"Not all evidence is created equal," George Wells said, as he began his overview of tools for assessing the quality of evidence from individual studies and systematic reviews. Based on an evaluation of many of the hundreds of available quality assessment instruments (QAIs), Wells and colleagues selected one known as SIGN 50 to use for assessing both randomized controlled trials (RCTs) and observational studies, but they believed that a nutrition-specific QAI would be even more sensitive to identifying bias in nutrition studies in particular. He explained how, using SIGN 50 as a starting point, they developed their own nutrition-specific QAI guidance for use by Health Canada. Among the many available instruments for quality assessment of nutrition studies at the systematic level review, Wells remarked that probably the most widely used for RCTs is AMSTAR, published in 2007. He noted that an updated AMSTAR2 for use with nonrandomized studies in addition to RCTs, and thus of relevance to the types of reviews being discussed at this workshop, will be the latest QAI tool to the marketplace.

"We have arrived at a stage in which the use and usefulness of systematic reviews to inform nutrition decisions are no longer debated," Joseph Lau claimed. This was not true 10–15 years ago. Lau explained the value

BOX 5-1
Overview of Points Presented by Individual Speakers

- A nutrition-specific quality assessment instrument (QAI) was developed for use by Health Canada to assess the quality of evidence from individual nutrition studies. The most widely used tool used for assessing the quality of systematic reviews is AMSTAR, but it can only be used for randomized controlled trials (RCTs). However, an updated AMSTAR2 will soon be available for use with nonrandomized studies in addition to RCTs, and thus of relevance to the types of reviews discussed at this workshop (Wells).
- The use and usefulness of systematic reviews to inform nutrition decisions are no longer debated. However, in the United States, if conducted through the Evidence-based Practice Centers Program of the Agency for Healthcare Research and Quality (AHRQ), a review may cost anywhere from $300,000 to $500,000. The use of a predefined analytic framework helps clarify systematic review questions (Lau).
- Risk–benefit assessment is a useful tool for estimating the public health burden associated with risk of inadequacy (at low intake levels) or risk of an adverse effect (at high intake levels). However, the work of scientists is limited to describing risk–benefit relationships. It is the policy makers who decide what to do with the information (Verhagen).

of using a predefined analytic framework to help clarify systematic review questions, using his work with vitamin D as an example. Additionally, he described several available resources to facilitate global harmonization of systematic review methods, including standards for conducting systematic reviews (e.g., *Cochrane Handbook for Systematic Review of Interventions*) and Web-based collaborative systematic review tools such as the open-access Systematic Review Data Repository (SRDR). In closing, Lau emphasized the likelihood that different countries may need to convene their own expert panels to develop nutrient intake recommendations but with the different panels using the same systematic reviews. As he put it, "Evidence is global, decision is local."

In the final presentation of this session, Hans Verhagen used past work with folic acid to illustrate how risk–benefit assessment can be used to estimate the public health burden associated with risk of inadequacy (at low intake levels) and/or risk of an adverse effect (at high intake levels). He and colleagues modeled the public health burden of folic acid fortification of flour at different doses and found that fortification would have both benefits and risks, including a decreased incidence of neural tube defects and an increased incidence of masked vitamin B12 deficiency. The potential public health burden associated with risk of colorectal cancer was less clear, according to Verhagen. Overall, their results suggested that a moderate level of fortification would decrease the public health burden associated with folic acid intake. Verhagen emphasized, however, that the work of scientists is to describe risk–benefit relationships, in contrast to the work of policy makers which is to do something with that information. In fact, he noted, the government decided not to fortify with folic acid, but to supplement instead.

TOOLS FOR EVALUATING STRENGTH AND QUALITY OF EVIDENCE[1]

George Wells began by commenting on the presentations he had heard thus far and the studies discussed. "All of them go back to the evidence itself," he said. "Not all evidence is created equal."

Evaluating Evidence at the Individual Study Level

At the individual study level, in order to obtain information about an intervention or exposure, there needs to be a comparison, Wells explained. This comparison can be made using any of a number of different study designs: experimental, including RCTs; quasi-experimental; or observational, including cohort, case-control, and cross-sectional studies (Reeves et al., 2017). He agreed with Amanda MacFarlane that observational studies will likely be the mainstay of future harmonization work around chronic disease endpoints (a summary of MacFarlane's presentation is included in Chapter 3).

All of these different types of studies can be arranged into a levels-of-evidence hierarchy, with RCTs generally providing the strongest evidence and therefore occupying the top tier (see Figure 3-1 from MacFarlane's presentation). Quasi-experimental studies occupy the next lowest tier, followed by cohort studies, then case-control studies, and cross-sectional studies at the bottom. The interesting feature of this evidence pyramid, Wells opined, is that, even within each tier there are different levels of quality of evidence depending on specific design features and conduct. "Different things can go wrong," he said, with "thousands and hundreds" of biases that can affect a study.

Biases can affect a study at any point along the course of events that occur during a study, as illustrated in Figure 5-1. Wells categorized these biases into seven "buckets," or domains, two of which can occur before an intervention, one at the time of intervention, and the other four after an

[1] This section summarizes information presented by George Wells, Ph.D., director, Cardiovascular Research Methods Centre, University of Ottawa, Ontario, Canada.

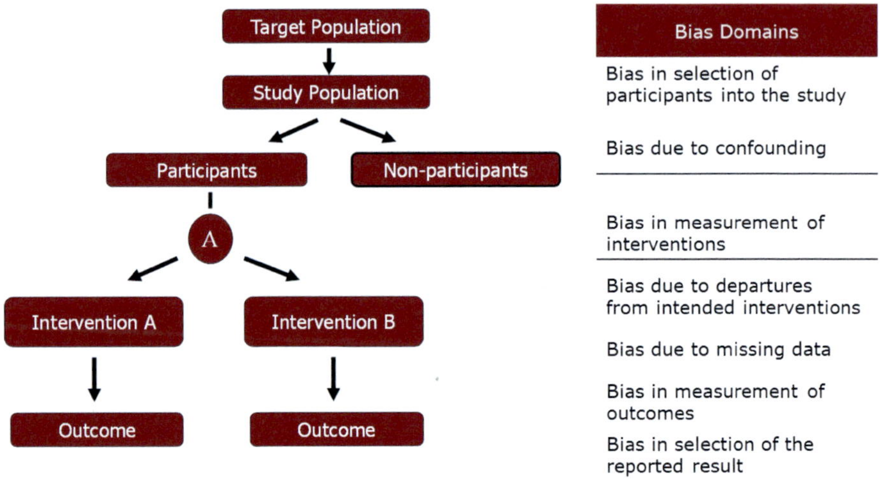

FIGURE 5-1 A flow chart of events that occur during a study, with the seven different types of biases that can occur along the way. The list of biases are aligned with where in a study they occur (e.g., selection bias occurs during the selection of participants versus nonparticipants, bias attributable to missing data occurs when outcomes are measured).
SOURCE: Presented by George Wells, HMD Workshop, Rome, Italy, September 21, 2017 (reprinted with permission).

intervention or exposure. Each of these buckets contains a number of different biases, he clarified. The selection bias bucket, for example, is not just selection bias, but also includes allocation bias, case mix bias, channeling bias, and so forth. Of interest, he noted, is that the four biases that occur after an intervention has been assigned can operate in both randomized and nonrandomized study designs. The other three biases are not an issue for well-designed RCTs, only for observational studies.

The Use of QAIs to Evaluate Bias

One way to evaluate the quality of evidence of individual studies, Wells continued, is through the use of QAIs. There are hundreds of such instruments. In a 2012 review, he and colleagues (Bai et al., 2012) identified 94 QAIs for RCTs, of which 32 reached a second-level evaluation. Of those 32, Bai et al. (2012) identified SIGN 50 as the most appropriate QAI. Similarly, they identified 99 QAIs for observational studies, of which 23 reached the second-level evaluation. Of those 23, they selected, again, SIGN 50.

Wells explained that the SIGN 50 methodological checklist for RCTs contains 10 items for what SIGN 50 calls "internal validity." These 10 items address, for example, how participants were randomized, how they were concealed, and whether the assessment was done in a blinded fashion. After looking at these items, rather than assigning a number or some sort of grade, an overall assessment is made based on which of the criteria were met. If the majority of criteria were met and the results unlikely to be changed by future research, then internal validity receives a "high-quality" rating. If most criteria were met, but there were some flaws in the study with an associated risk of bias such that the conclusions of the study may change in light of further studies, then the study receives an "acceptable" rating. However, if either most criteria were not met or there were significant flaws relating to critical aspects of the study design, such that the conclusions are likely to change in light of future research, then the study receives a "low-quality" rating. In addition to the actual assessment questions, the SIGN 50 instrument also provides guidance for answering each question, Wells noted. Similarly, for case-control and cohort studies, an overall assessment is made after assessing each criterion separately. "It is a well-used approach," Wells said.

Although he did not delve into the details of how Bai et al. (2012) conducted their review, Wells did note that very few of the 32 RCT QAIs that reached the second-level evaluation fully satisfied the seven criteria used to evaluate them (i.e., study population, randomization, blinding, interventions, outcomes, statistical analysis, funding). Similarly for the observational studies, very few of the 23 that reached the second-level evaluation fully satisfied the five criteria used to evaluate them (i.e., comparability of subjects, exposure/intervention, outcome measure, statistical analysis, funding).

In addition to QAIs, Bai et al. (2012) also evaluated evidence grading systems and selected, among the 60 identified and 23 that made it to the second-level evaluation, the Grading of Recommendations Assessment, Development and Evaluation (GRADE) approach.

Health Canada's Nutrition-Specific QAI Project

MacFarlane and her colleagues at Health Canada, along with Wells and his colleagues at the University of Ottawa, were currently (at the time of this workshop) working on developing a nutrition-specific QAI. The genesis of this work was the "Options Report" (Yetley et al., 2016). It became quite apparent during that process, Wells recalled, that the existing QAIs were not sensitive enough to evaluate nutrition evidence relating to chronic disease endpoints for Dietary Reference Intakes (DRIs), nor were they sensitive enough to determine which studies had high bias versus low bias. He and others felt that a nutrition-specific QAI would be useful, as it would be made more sensitive by taking into account the specific covariates, confounders, and sources of error unique to nutrition.

Wells described in detail the seven critical steps he and his Health Canada and University of Ottawa colleagues have taken to develop a nutrition-specific QAI. First, they established some general development principles. They wanted to conduct the process in a simple way that allowed them to incorporate components of nutrition studies that would make the tool more sensitive. They decided they would do this through what Wells called "bolt on." That is, they would "bolt on" to an existing QAI-specific question related to nutrition. They would also build guidance for the nutrition-specific questions, similar to the guidance that existed for the SIGN 50 internal validity questions. They planned to borrow all of the same psychometric properties of the original QAI.

Second, they needed to identify which QAI to use. According to Wells, upon examining the newest literature, their opinion about SIGN 50 did not change (i.e., based on their Bai et al. [2012] review of QAIs), and they decided to use it.

Third, they conducted a scoping review to identify which nutrition-specific appraisal items to include in the new tool, building on the seven nutrition-specific items proposed by Chung et al. (2009a) to consider based on the concern that failure to consider these items could lead to a biased synthesis or interpretation of results in a nutrient-related systematic review. There was then some discussion about the items in Washington, DC, and then a panel was convened to refine the list of proposed items.

Fourth, they decided on five nutrition-specific items for RCTs, five for cohort studies, and two for case-control studies. Specifically, for RCTs, they decided, first, that the relevant intake nutritional status at baseline should be documented and taken into account. Second, they decided that the background intakes of all groups should be maintained over the course of the study. Third, they decided that the amount of intervention intake under study should be quantitatively measured and the form, where relevant, described. Fourth, adherence to the intervention and control intakes should be monitored in a reliable and accurate manner. And fifth, the interval between intervention and outcome should be of sufficient duration to observe an effect if there is an effect to observe. The five items for cohort studies were similar, Wells said.

The fifth step in their development of a nutrition-specific QAI was to format the questions. For RCTs, for example, they kept the same general quality appraisal items as the original SIGN 50 QAI and then, Wells said, they "bolted on" the nutrition-specific items. They did the same for cohort and case-control studies.

Sixth, they developed guidance for completing the questionnaire for each newly added item. Adding guidance was an important part of the process, Wells emphasized. Failure to provide good guidance is, he said, "usually the failure of these types of instruments."

Finally, they conducted a reliability and validity check. They selected 10 published studies of RCTs of nutrient-health outcomes and asked two independent reviewers to apply the newly developed QAI for RCTs to each of these 10 studies. Wells explained that the purpose of this step was to evaluate the reliability of the reviewers' assessments, determine validity of the QAI, and identify the effect of the additional information provided by the nutrition-specific items. They did the same for the cohort and case-control QAIs.

The end result of this process is illustrated in Figure 5-2, although only the item checklist and overall assessment portions are shown, not the accompanying guidance. The guidance took an enormous amount of time to develop, Wells remarked. It includes both overall information on assessing intake and nutritional status, as well as several other concepts, plus information for each individual question.

According to Wells, the status of this project (at the time of the workshop) was that both the forms and guidance had been developed for RCTs, case-control, and cohort studies. In addition, for the RCT QAI, testing had

SIGN

Methodology Checklist 2: Controlled Trials

Study identification (*Include author, title, year of publication, journal title, pages*)

Guideline topic:	Key Question No:	Reviewer:

Before completing this checklist, consider:

1. Is the paper a **randomised controlled trial** or a **controlled clinical trial**? If in doubt, check the study design algorithm available from SIGN and make sure you have the correct checklist. If it is a **controlled clinical trial** questions 1.2, 1.3, and 1.4 are not relevant, and the study cannot be rated higher than 1+
2. Is the paper relevant to key question? Analyse using PICO (Patient or Population Intervention Comparison Outcome). IF NO REJECT (give reason below). IF YES complete the checklist.

Reason for rejection: 1. Paper not relevant to key question ☐ 2. Other reason ☐ (please specify):

SECTION 1: INTERNAL VALIDITY

	In a well conducted RCT study…	***Does this study do it?***
1.1	The study addresses an appropriate and clearly focused question.	Yes ☐ No ☐ Can't say ☐
1.2	The assignment of subjects to treatment groups is randomised.	Yes ☐ No ☐ Can't say ☐
1.3	An adequate concealment method is used.	Yes ☐ No ☐ Can't say ☐
1.4	The design keeps subjects and investigators 'blind' about treatment allocation.	Yes ☐ No ☐ Can't say ☐
1.5	The treatment and control groups are similar at the start of the trial.	Yes ☐ No ☐ Can't say ☐
1.6	The only difference between groups is the treatment under investigation.	Yes ☐ No ☐ Can't say ☐
1.7	All relevant outcomes are measured in a standard, valid and reliable way.	Yes ☐ No ☐ Can't say ☐
1.8	What percentage of the individuals or clusters recruited into each treatment arm of the study dropped out before the study was completed?	
1.9	All the subjects are analysed in the groups to which they were randomly allocated (often referred to as intention to treat analysis).	Yes ☐ No ☐ Can't say ☐ Does not apply ☐
1.10	Where the study is carried out at more than one site, results are comparable for all sites.	Yes ☐ No ☐ Can't say ☐ Does not apply ☐

SECTION 2: INTERNAL VALIDITY - NUTRITION SPECIFIC ASPECTS

	In a well-conducted nutrition RCT study…	***Does this study do it?***
2.1	The relevant intake/nutritional status at baseline is sufficiently documented.	Yes ☐ No ☐ Can't say ☐
2.2	The baseline intakes of all groups have been maintained over the course of the study.	Yes ☐ No ☐ Can't say ☐
2.3	The amount of intervention intake under study has been quantitatively measured and the form, where relevant, has been described.	Yes ☐ No ☐ Can't say ☐
2.4	Adherence to the intervention and control intakes is being monitored in a reliable and accurate manner.	Yes ☐ No ☐ Can't say ☐
2.5	The interval between the intervention and outcome is of sufficient duration to observe an effect, if there is one.	Yes ☐ No ☐ Can't say ☐

SECTION 3: OVERALL ASSESSMENT OF THE STUDY

3.1	How well was the study done to minimize bias? When making your overall assessment of the design and analysis of the study, take into consideration the importance and relevance of each of the preceding 15 items as it relates to your research question and weight it in your overall assessment accordingly. The rationale for the assessment strategy should be documented.	High quality (++)☐ Acceptable (+)☐ Unacceptable – reject 0 ☐
3.2	Taking into account clinical/population health considerations, your evaluation of the methodology used, and the statistical power of the study, are you certain that the overall effect is due to the study intervention?	
3.3	Are the results of this study directly applicable to the patient/population group targeted by this guideline?	
3.4	**Notes.** Summarize the authors' conclusions. Add any comments on your own assessment of the study, and the extent to which it answers your question and mention any areas of uncertainty raised above.	

FIGURE 5-2 The nutrition-specific quality assessment instrument (QAI) developed by Wells and colleagues for Health Canada with the same internal validity checklist as in the original SIGN 50 QAI, plus the newly developed nutrition-specific section and a revised overall assessment section.

SOURCES: Presented by George Wells, HMD Workshop, Rome, Italy, September 21, 2017 (adapted from SIGN, 2015).

been completed, and modifications were being made. The cohort and case-control QAIs were still being tested. Manuscripts were also being prepared for submission.

Risk of Bias

Today, the current trend when examining quality of evidence is to examine risk of bias, Wells continued. The difference between risk-of-bias instruments and QAIs is subtle, he said. Risk of bias usually involves examining one particular outcome and anything that can go wrong that will shift the estimate of that outcome; whereas, QAIs are more like quality appraisals. That is, they examine how explicit and transparent the methods are and apply the rules of evidence to factors such as internal validity, adherence to reporting standards, conclusions, and generalizability. In his opinion, there is a need for both types of tools.

As an example of a risk-of-bias tool being used to evaluate RCTs, Wells mentioned the Cochrane Risk of Bias Tool, included in the *Cochrane Handbook for Systematic Reviews of Interventions* ("the Cochrane handbook") (Higgins and Green, 2011). The tool assesses six domains of bias, judging each as low, unclear, or high risk.

An example of a risk-of-bias tool being used to evaluate nonrandomized studies is the ROBINS-1 tool (Sterne et al., 2016). It is a little bit more involved, Wells remarked, and difficult to fill out. It would be particularly difficult to fill out for a systematic review. In his opinion, its best use may be for individual observational studies. It includes the seven bias domains mentioned previously and listed in Figure 5-1, with signaling questions pertaining to each particular bias. Signaling questions, Wells explained, are factual questions that lead the user to respond "yes," "possibly yes," "possibly no," or "no." There is also free text to help users decide their answers. Then, an assessment of each bias is made by looking across all the signaling questions for that bias. One can also examine the direction of each bias. Finally, by combining all the biases, one can make a judgment about the overall risk of bias as either low, moderate, serious, or critical.

Evaluating Evidence at the Systematic Review Level

At the systematic review level, one could collate and assemble into summary tables or figures all of the QAIs and risk-of-bias assessments for all of the individual studies. Wells showed a couple of what he considered classical examples of these summary tables and figures from the Cochrane handbook. Or, one could use a measurement instrument known as AMSTAR to assess the methodological quality of the review. In the Bai et al. (2012) review of QAIs, AMSTAR was selected as the most appropriate QAI for systematic reviews. Although AMSTAR is widely used (Shea et al., 2007), it was not designed to handle nonrandomized studies.

An updated AMSTAR2 that will allow for evaluation of nonrandomized studies, in addition to RCTs, will be the latest QAI tool to the marketplace, according to Wells. Described in Shea et al. (2017), AMSTAR2 was developed by a global group. The tool asks about study selection and data exclusion, risk of bias, sources of funding, inclusion of nonrandomized studies, issues around heterogeneity, and other items.

Next Steps

Wells summarized several recent developments: the Reeves et al. (2017) taxonomy of individual level studies (i.e., experimental, quasi-experimental, and observational); publication of AMSTAR2 (Shea et al., 2017), which, because it will cover nonrandomized studies, will be important for the types of reviews being discussed at this workshop, Wells predicted; and the ROBINS-1 risk-of-bias tool, which was specifically designed for nonrandomized studies and thus, again, is relevant to harmonization, in Wells's opinion.

Currently in development, but ready soon, is the nutrition-specific QAI that Wells and colleagues have been developing for RCTs, cohort studies, and case-control studies (i.e., the SIGN 50 bolt-on). Also currently in development is a nutrition-specific QAI for cross-sectional studies, which will be analogous to the SIGN 50 QAI, but requires more than a simple "bolt-on;" and a revised risk-of-bias tool for RCTs (i.e., by the Bristol Appraisal and Review of Research group at the University of Bristol, United Kingdom).

Finally, in planning are de novo (i.e., not bolt-on) nutrition-specific QAIs for RCTs, cohort studies, case-control studies, and cross-sectional studies; a nutrition-specific risk-of-bias tool (i.e., a bolt-on tool); and a nutrition-specific tool for evaluating systematic reviews (i.e., an AMSTAR2 bolt-on).

In conclusion, Wells reflected on a lesson learned from his involvement in these recent and current developments, which is the value of developing a nutrition-specific QAI from the start (i.e., not as a bolt-on). Such a tool may take longer to develop, he said, but it could streamline the actual evaluation process. Evaluating a nutritional intervention is not the same as developing a drug or device.

GLOBAL SYSTEMATIC REVIEWS: HOW CAN IT BE DONE?[2]

Joseph Lau began his talk by listing four assumptions. First, he said, "We have arrived at a stage in which the use and usefulness of systematic review to inform nutrition decisions is no longer debated." This was not true 10 to 15 years ago. Second, much of what has been learned about the methods and processes of systematic reviews comes from the health care arena, but that knowledge can be applied to the nutrition world. "We should try to minimize reinventing the wheel whenever possible," he said. Third, evidence is global, but decisions are local. "Because we are all human," he explained, the same evidence can be used to inform nutrient intake recommendations. Finally, conducting a systematic review is laborious and requires a significant amount of resources, including expertise, time, and money; thus, it is desirable to minimize replication of effort and to collaborate and share resources. Lau then went on to discuss systematic reviews in detail, beginning with the importance of such reviews and the value of a harmonized systematic review protocol.

Applying Systematic Reviews and a Harmonized Protocol to Review Evidence

In a 2005 World Health Organization (WHO)/Food and Agriculture Organization (FAO) report on nutrient risk assessment, Lau and Alice Lichtenstein contributed a discussion paper titled "Evidence-Based Approach to Nutrient Hazard Identification" (WHO/FAO, 2005). At that time, Lau recalled, there was growing international interest in the use of nutrient risk assessment to identify the tolerable upper level of intake (UL) for nutrients and related substance, but also recognition of the need for a common approach. Different authoritative bodies had come up with different ULs, including for vitamin A (i.e., in relation to bone health), which Lau and Lichtenstein were asked to use as an example in their paper. The U.S. Institute of Medicine (IOM) recommended (in 2001) 3,000 micrograms of vitamin A per day (μg/d) for adults; the European Union (EU) Scientific Committee on Food recommended (in 2002) that postmenopausal women restrict their intake to 1,500 μg/d; and the United Kingdom (UK) Expert Group in Vitamins & Minerals suggested (in 2003) that daily total intake should not exceed 1,500 μg/d.

Lau and Lichtenstein compared the evidence that these different groups had examined, the questions they had asked, and the methodologies they applied. For example, Lau described how they categorized the approxi-

---

[2] This section summarizes information presented by Joseph Lau, M.D., professor, Center for Evidence-based Medicine, School of Public Health, Brown University, Providence, Rhode Island.

mately 30 references used in the three reports to justify or support their recommendations by type of study: in vitro (e.g., cell or bone culture), animal, or human. They found that the EU study cited many of all three types of studies, the UK report cited several animal studies and many human studies, and the U.S. report cited mostly human studies and one animal study. Thus, different work groups used different sets of studies. Moreover, Lau added, none described how they selected their studies, that is, what their inclusion/exclusion criteria were, or how the included studies were used to support their recommendations.

Based on their examination, Lau and Lichtenstein concluded the following:

- Lack of a preanalytical framework affected the selection of specific outcomes to assess evidence.
- Lack of a common set of research questions and review criteria led to the selection of different studies.
- Use of different types of studies (i.e., in vitro, animal, human) and the different emphasis placed on the evidence might have led to different interpretations of the data and characterization of the hazard.
- The composition of the work groups may have been different, with different groups of experts weighing evidence differently (e.g., one group may have had more toxicologists than another).

A Representative Systematic Review Process

To illustrate a representative systematic review process, Lau described the "evidence report" employed by the Agency for Healthcare Research and Quality (AHRQ) for the past 20 years. The process involves five main steps:

1. Prepare the topic—refine questions and develop an analytic framework
2. Search for and select studies—identify eligibility criteria, search for relevant studies, and select evidence for inclusion
3. Abstract data—extract evidence from studies and construct evidence tables
4. Analyze and synthesize data—assess quality of studies, assess applicability of studies, apply qualitative methods, apply quantitative methods such as meta-analysis, and rate the strength of a body of evidence
5. Present findings

Not included in this list of steps, Lau pointed out, are identifying a systematic review team, forming a technical expert panel, and performing peer review of the draft report. Importantly, he added, the end product, the evidence report itself, does not constitute either clinical or policy recommendations. "It is just information," he said, that is interpreted and used by the appropriate committee to draft recommendations.

A well-conducted systematic review takes about 1 year, according to Lau. The literature search, which includes both the screening of abstracts and extracting data from primary articles, occupies the largest amount of time (i.e., 6 months of a year-long review). Another large amount of time is spent on peer review and revision of the draft paper. In the United States, if conducted through the Evidence-based Practice Centers (EPCs) Program of the AHRQ, a review may cost anywhere from $300,000 to $500,000.

The Use of an Analytic Framework to Help Identify Systematic Review Questions

Lau emphasized the value of using an analytic framework (e.g., a causal pathway) to clarify and generate systematic review questions. Constructing such a framework involves formulating and organizing relevant questions into a model that analyzes all the effects and interactions between intervention or exposure and outcomes (see Figure 5-3). The value of such a framework, Lau explained, is that it helps to define the scope of the evidence and to construct an evidence map of the many questions that potentially could be addressed. "It gives you the lay of land of the literature to see whether a systematic review is even possible," Lau said. If there is not enough evidence, then money should not be invested in a systematic review; on the other hand, if there is too much evidence, one should probably find a way to reduce the scope of the work. It is valuable in other ways as well, Lau continued: It uses experts efficiently; the framework and process can be open to public review, thereby providing transparency and minimizing biases; it can help to highlight what aspects are known and unknown; it can clarify which study designs (e.g., experimental or observational) may be best to address specific questions; and it can be used to facilitate future updates of systematic reviews as new evidence emerges.

As an example of how an analytic framework has been used to inform DRI development, Lau described the framework he and his team at Tufts University provided to IOM in 2009 for vitamin D and/or calcium and associated health outcomes (see Figure 5-4). Lau noted the framework also captured ultraviolet exposure and that an expert panel was convened to help define which health outcomes to study. A strategic question in the framework (illustrated by arrow 1 in Figure 5-4) was: What is the effect of vitamin D, calcium, or combined vitamin D and calcium intake on clinical

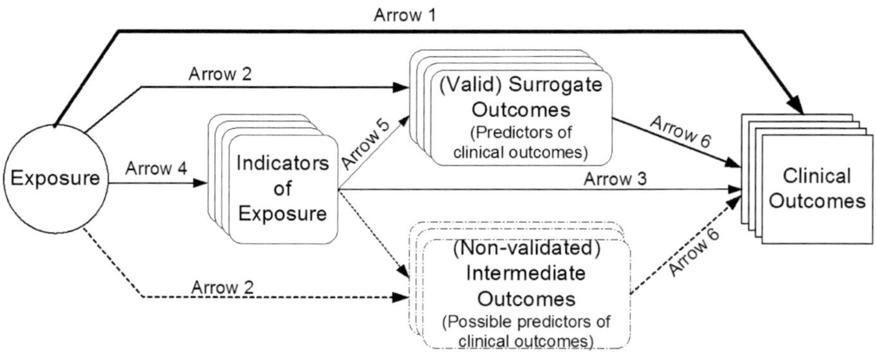

FIGURE 5-3 Generic analytic framework for a systematic review of studies on the associations between a nutrient and health outcomes. Arrow 1: association of exposure with clinical outcomes of interest. Arrow 2: association of exposure with surrogate or intermediate outcomes. Arrow 3: association of indicators of exposure to clinical outcomes Arrow 4: association between exposure and indicators of exposure. Arrow 5: association of indicators of exposure to surrogate or intermediate outcomes. Arrow 6: association between surrogate outcomes and clinical outcomes.
SOURCES: Presented by Joseph Lau, HMD Workshop, Rome, Italy, September 21, 2017 (reprinted with permission, Russell et al., 2009).

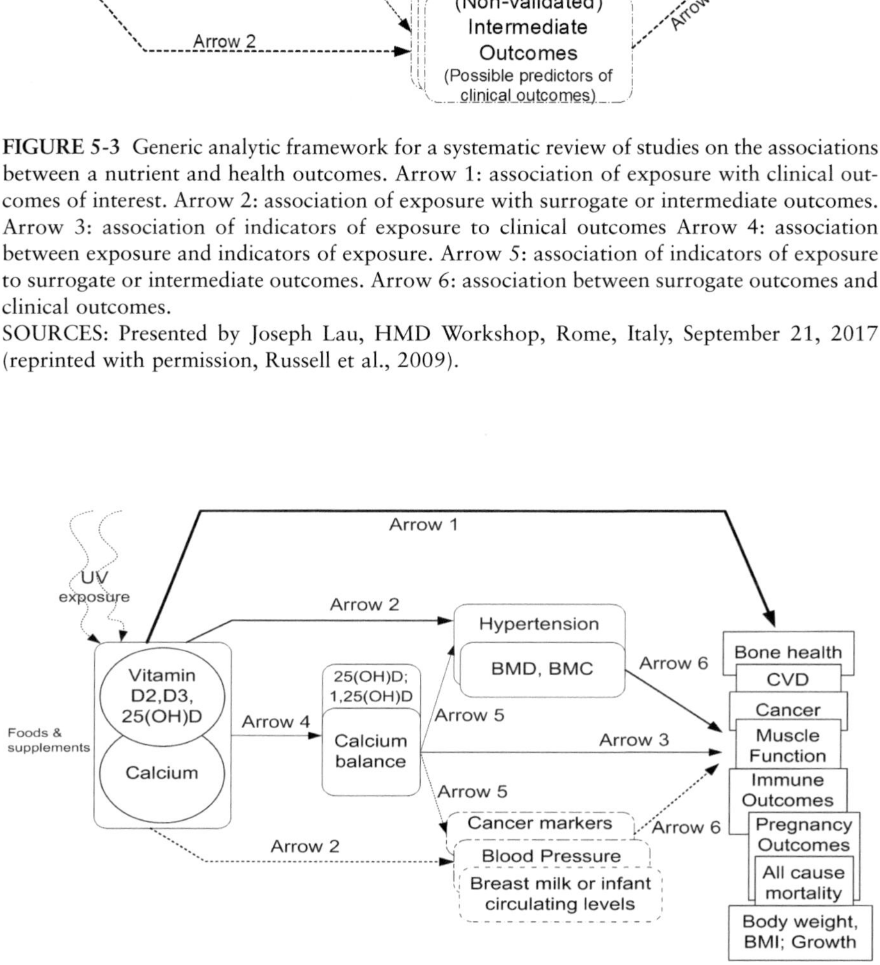

FIGURE 5-4 Analytic framework for vitamin D and/or calcium and associated health outcomes.
NOTE: BMC = bone mineral content; BMD = bone mineral density; BMI = body mass index; CVD = cardiovascular disease; UV = ultraviolet radiation.
SOURCES: Presented by Joseph Lau, HMD Workshop, Rome, Italy, September 21, 2017 (reprinted with permission, Chung et al., 2009b).

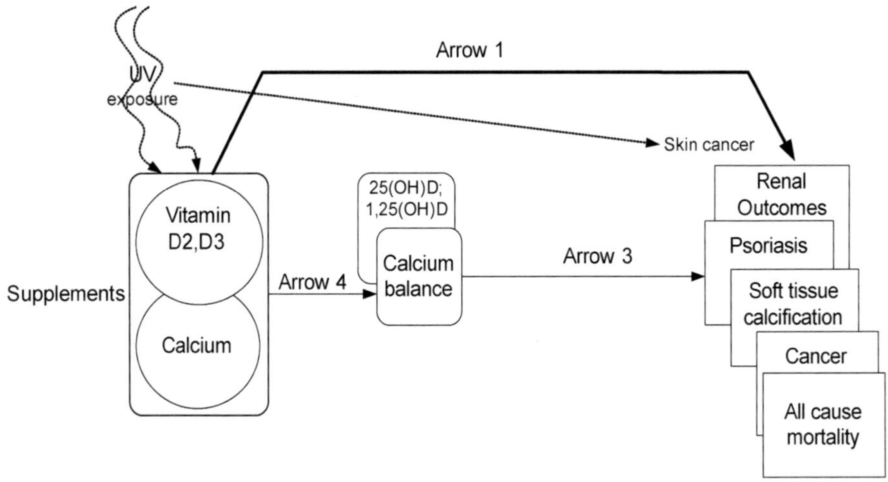

FIGURE 5-5 Analytic framework for vitamin D and/or calcium and associated safety-related (adverse) outcomes.
SOURCES: Presented by Joseph Lau, HMD Workshop, Rome, Italy, September 21, 2017 (reprinted with permission, Chung et al., 2009b).

outcomes, including growth, cardiovascular diseases, weight outcomes, cancer, immune function, pregnancy or birth outcomes, mortality, fracture, renal outcomes, and soft tissue calcification? A second question (illustrated by arrow 2 in Figure 5-4) was: What is the effect of vitamin D, calcium, or combined vitamin D and calcium on surrogate or intermediate outcomes, such as hypertension, blood pressure, and bone mineral density? Additionally, a separate analytic framework was constructed for safety-related outcomes related to the UL, as illustrated in Figure 5-5.

Using these two analytic frameworks, a technical expert panel specified the PICOS (population, interventions/exposures, comparators, and outcomes of interest) selection criteria for each question. Of this step in general, Lau said that it "could be very involved." He shared a partial list of the PICOS criteria specified for the vitamin D and/or calcium frameworks. For example, the population criteria included generally healthy people with no known disorders, studies that enrolled fewer than 20 percent of patients with common diseases, and any population for adverse effects of high intake. The outcome criteria included 17 outcomes selected by the technical expert panel.

With this information, the systematic review team was then able to conduct its literature search. They reviewed more than 16,000 primary study citations and ended up selecting 165 of these, plus some additional systematic reviews. Specifically, they identified 16,733 citations in a MEDLINE and Cochrane Central database search for primary studies published between 1969 and April 2009, and 1,746 citations in a MEDLINE, Cochrane Database of Systematic Reviews, and the Health Technology Assessments database search for systematic review articles published before December 2008. Of these, they retrieved 584 primary study articles for full-text review and 68 systematic review articles for full-text review. Of these, they reviewed 165 primary study articles (60 RCTs, 3 nonrandomized controlled trials, and 102 cohort or case-control studies) and 11 systematic reviews.

Without going into detail regarding the specifics of the 2009 vitamin D/calcium review, Lau explained that, after a literature search and selection is completed, the next step is to report the evidence. Data are extracted from each study and entered into evidence tables and summaries of each study (i.e., outcomes, study design) are entered into summary tables. From these, figures and graphs can be constructed. Additionally, meta-analyses can be conducted, if appropriate. A narrative, highlighting features and limitations of the review in answering the question, is also included. Finally, Lau reiterated that an evidence report in itself does not make recommendations.

Global Harmonization of Systematic Reviews

Several resources are available to facilitate the global harmonization of systematic reviews. First among these are standards that exist for the conduct of a systematic review. Lau mentioned AHRQ's very detailed *Methods Guide for Effectiveness and Comparative Effectiveness Reviews* (AHRQ, 2008–2017); Cochrane's *Handbook for Systematic Review of Interventions*, also a very detailed manual, he noted (Higgins and Green, 2011); and the IOM's 2011 *Finding What Works in Health Care: Standards for Systematic Reviews* (IOM, 2011b). There are also standards for reporting systematic reviews and meta-analyses. Additionally, although not part of a review of evidence, Lau mentioned standards for clinical practice guidelines.

In addition to these standards, there are several Web-based collaborative systematic review tools that could be helpful to facilitating a harmonized approach. One of these is the SRDR (srdr.ahrq.gov), of which Lau disclosed that he had been the director since 2010. He described the depository as an open access systematic review tool that can be used collaboratively. It creates data abstraction forms, collects data, produces reports, and interfaces with other systematic review tools, such as the Data Abstraction Assistant. Users voluntarily contribute and share data used in systematic reviews so the data can be reused for updated reviews and so the transparency of the systematic review process is improved. The SRDR was developed and is currently (at the time of this workshop) maintained by Brown University's EPC. Launched in 2012, the depository also involves an international governance board.

The Structure of a Systematic Review

Based on the recently released National Academies report *Redesigning the Process for Establishing the* Dietary Guidelines for Americans (NASEM, 2017b), Lau offered some suggestions on structure for ensuring high-quality systematic reviews. First among these is that there should be an oversight body to provide strategic direction. This could be the sponsor, he noted. Second, already there are what are known as nutrient intake recommendation committees, which make recommendations informed by systematic reviews. Some of these committee members, Lau suggested, should be part of the technical expert panel. Third, the technical expert panel assists the systematic review team in refining critical questions and helps to develop review criteria. Importantly, Lau emphasized, to minimize bias, members of the technical expert panel should not participate in the actual systematic review. Fourth, the systematic review team should be a group that independently carries out the systematic review once a protocol has been developed. Finally, all reviews should be reviewed by peers.

Regarding membership on a systematic review team, Lau cited *Finding What Works in Health Care: Standards for Systematic Reviews* (IOM, 2011b), where it was stated that the teams should be multidisciplinary and include methodologists, content experts, librarians or information scientists, statisticians, and additional members as needed, such as editors and research assistants, and that members should be free of conflict of interest.

Closing Thoughts

Lau shared several closing thoughts. First, he said, "Evidence is not static." Nutrient intake recommendations may need to be updated. Thus, there is a need to monitor new evidence and to have a process for updating systematic reviews and nutrient intake recommendations. Second, repeating one of his opening statements that evidence is global, but decisions are local, he suggested that different countries convene their own expert panels to come up with nutrient intake recommendations, using the same framework and evidence base but incorporating local dietary patterns and other factors. Third, he emphasized that his presentation focused on the synthesis of evidence, not on decision making around recommendations. Finally, he emphasized the importance of separating tasks and using separate expert groups to review the evidence and interpret the results.

RISK–BENEFIT ASSESSMENT OF FOODS IN A EUROPEAN PERSPECTIVE[3]

Across the globe, it is believed that "food should be safe," Hans Verhagen began. Yet, humans are inclined to take risks, he said. Some people dare to smoke, some buy lottery tickets or stock shares, while others practice dietary habits that are not fully compatible with dietary recommendations. He elaborated, "We are inclined to take risks if we get something out of it—something better."

Before presenting his overview of risk–benefit assessment in relation to nutrition and food safety, using his past work at the Netherlands National Institute for Public Health and the Environment (RIVM) with folic acid as an example, Verhagen noted that the European Food Safety Authority (EFSA) has done considerable work in the area of dietary reference values (DRVs), with DRVs for only three nutrients still outstanding (chloride, sodium, sugars). He referred workshop participants to EFSA's recently published summary report of completed DRV reports (EFSA, 2017a). Additionally, in 2006, EFSA completed an overview of ULs established by either EFSA or its predecessor, the EU Scientific Committee for Food. Those UL values are still valid today, with only a few updates having been proposed since 2006.

Dietary Reference Values: Risk–Benefit Assessment

To illustrate risk–benefit assessment, Verhagen considered a hypothetical micronutrient and a population distribution of daily intake for that nutrient. As shown in Figure 5-6a, where the average intake of this hypothetical micronutrient is 120 (units unspecified), there is a small percentage of people, say 5 percent, whose intake is low. "They may constitute a public health risk," Verhagen said. Because 5 percent of a population is a lot of people, policy makers might decide to do something to reduce the public health risk. For example, one might decide to increase intake through fortification or supplementation. But then, as shown in Figure 5-6b, while the initial public health risk will have been solved by increasing intake of the problem micronutrient, another problem will have been created: Now there is a small percentage of the population, in this example, 5 percent, whose intake is so high that, again, there is a public health risk. A combination of these two scenarios, Verhagen explained, illustrates risk–benefit (see Figure 5-6c).

---

[3] This section summarizes information presented by Hans Verhagen, Ph.D., head, Risk Assessment and Scientific Assistance Department, European Food Safety Authority (EFSA), Parma, Italy.

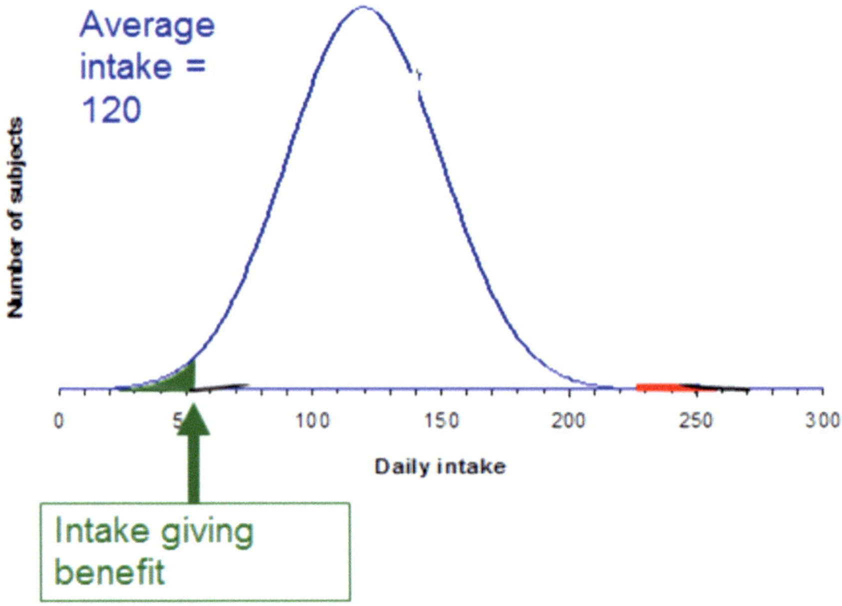

FIGURE 5-6A

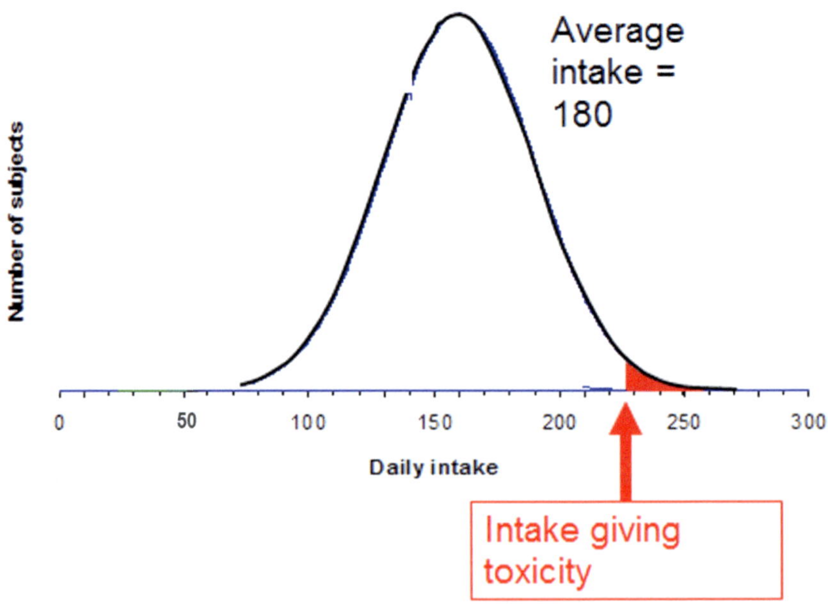

FIGURE 5-6B

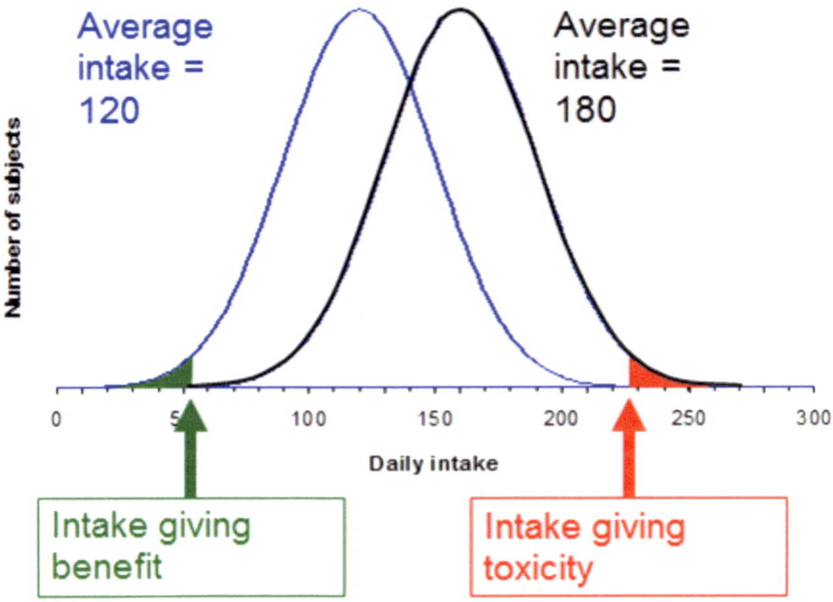

FIGURE 5-6C

FIGURE 5-6A–C Population distribution (y-axis) versus intake (x-axis; units unspecified) for a hypothetical nutrient. Subjects receiving daily intake below the "intake giving benefit" threshold are at risk because of their low intake (green area of curve); subjects receiving daily intake above the "intake giving toxicity" threshold are at risk because of their high intake (red area of curve).
SOURCE: Presented by Hans Verhagen, HMD Workshop, Rome, Italy, September 21, 2017.

Verhagen emphasized the difference between the role of the scientist in risk–benefit assessment versus the role of the policy maker. "As a scientist, you describe the curves," he said, referring to the curves in Figure 5-6, and "as a policy maker or politician, you make the decisions on the basis of the scientific information."

As an example of an actual nutrient risk–benefit assessment, Verhagen described his past work on folic acid, when he and colleagues at RIVM examined the huge database on folic acid in the literature (Hoekstra et al., 2007). They found, among the 30 to 40 potential effects reported, only a handful had sufficient evidence. Namely, they found that it is well established that folic acid can prevent neural tube defects. It is also well established that folic acid can also mask a vitamin B12 deficiency, typically in older age. A masked B12 deficiency, in turn, may lead to neurological damage that can be irreversible if maintained too long. Additionally, it is well established that folic acid can change the incidence of colorectal cancer, either increasing or decreasing it. Finally, folic acid intake can overcome a folate deficiency.

After identifying these handfuls of effects with well-established evidence, Hoekstra et al. (2007) used data from the Netherlands to calculate the expected public health effects of fortifying flour with different amounts of folic acid, from 70 micrograms (μg) through 420 μg per 100 grams (g). They found that, on a yearly basis, at 70 μg/100 g of flour, there would be 83 fewer incident cases of neural tube defects, amounting to a 37 percent decrease; an additional 53 people with masked vitamin B12 deficiencies, or a 1 percent increase; and 405 fewer cases of colorectal cancer, a 4.1 percent decrease. In terms of disability-adjusted life years (DALYs), neural tube defect DALYs would increase by 5,474, masked B12 deficiency DALYs would decrease by 53, and colorectal cancer DALYs would increase by 2,217, with many uncertainties.

Thus, the public health effects related to neural tube defects and colorectal cancer would represent a gain, but the effects related to masked B12 deficiency would be a loss. Additionally, for DALYs, Table 5-1 shows a clear dose–response relationship for all three effects, with the effects becoming more pronounced at higher fortification levels.

Verhagen emphasized that while there is a great deal of uncertainty especially around the colorectal cancer estimates shown in Table 5-1 a moderate fortification level of 70 μg would decrease the public health burden associated with folic acid intake. Additionally, he repeated that it is the scientists' job to present the evidence, but it is "at the discretion of the authorities to make a decision." In fact, the Netherlands government decided not to fortify in this case, but to supplement.

TABLE 5-1 Predicted Public Health Burden (DALYs) Associated with Different Levels of Flour Folic Acid Fortification

	Level of Folic Acid Fortification (micrograms [μg] per 100 g)			
	70	140	280	420
Neural tube defects	5,474	7,710	9,812	10,855
Masked B12 deficiency	–53	–76	–120	–165
Colorectal cancer	2,217	4,146	167	–21,740
Total	7,662	11,812	9,899	–11,006

SOURCES: Presented by Hans Verhagen, HMD Workshop, Rome, Italy, September 21, 2017 (Hoekstra et al., 2007, with permission from Elsevier).

Conducting Risk–Benefit Analysis: Things to Keep in Mind

When toxicologists think about risk–benefit, they think about it differently than nutritionists do, Verhagen continued. Toxicologists typically calculate things intended to not happen, he said. They do this by conducting animal studies and identifying no-observed-adverse-effect-levels (NOAELs) for food additives, pesticides, and other exposures. NOAELs are dose levels at and below which an effect no longer occurs. Then, so these values can be translated to humans, a safety factor is applied and an acceptable daily intake (ADI) determined. The ADI is an intake at which nothing happens. The safety factor is typically 100, and the ADI is typically two orders of magnitude below the NOAEL. According to Verhagen, this is the same thinking that is used to set safe ULs, although not by applying a safety factor of 100.

In contrast, he continued, "a nutritionist argues the other way around. In nutrition, we want something to happen." Rather than calculating the absence of an effect, a nutritionist calculates effects that will happen. This difference is illustrated in Figure 5-7, where a risk–benefit assessment of,

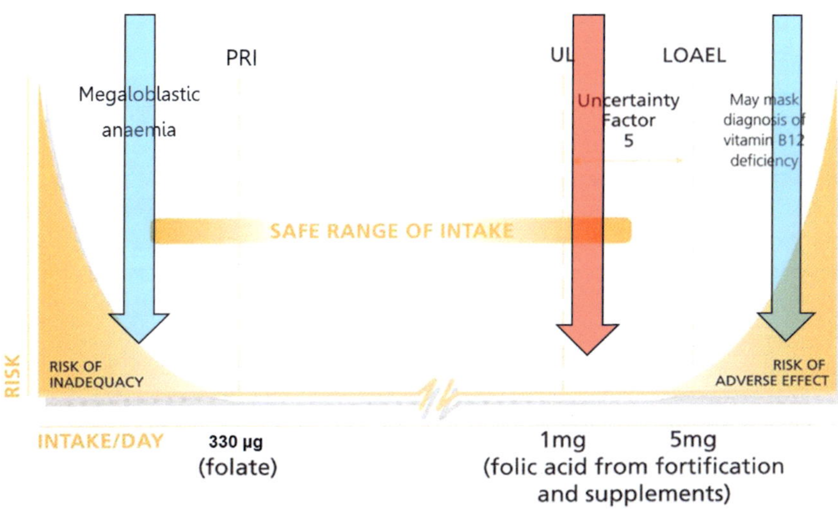

FIGURE 5-7 Risk–benefit curve showing risk of effects associated with deficient intake (represented by the blue arrow on the left), risk of adverse effects associated with excessive intake (represented by the blue arrow on the right), and the lack of risk associated with intake at the safe upper limit (middle, red arrow).
NOTE: LOAEL = lowest-observed-adverse-effect-level; PRI = population reference intake; UL = upper limit.
SOURCES: Presented by Hans Verhagen, HMD Workshop, Rome, Italy, September 21, 2017 (modified with permission, European Responsible Nutrition Alliance).

in this case, folic acid or folate requires comparing "risk of inadequacy" effects at the low end of the intake range (i.e., folate deficiency, neural tube defects) with "risk of adverse effect" effects at the high end (i.e., masking vitamin B12 deficiency). Too often, Verhagen said, people make comparisons with the UL, represented by the red arrow in the figure. But, again, the UL is set at a point at which nothing happens.

Verhagen mentioned several recently completed large risk–benefit assessment projects in Europe (i.e., Quality of Life–Integrated Benefit and Risk Analysis, Benefit–Risk Analysis for Foods, Benefit–Risk Analysis for Food: An Iterative Value-of-Information Approach, and Best Practices for Risk–Benefit Analysis), then posed the question, "What are the main outcomes of these big projects?" First, he said, "When doing risk–benefit, always think of at least two scenarios." For example, compare fortification with no fortification or sugar-sweetened beverages with artificially sweetened beverages. Second, use a common currency to describe the health effects. It could be DALYs, deaths, incident cases, or euros spent on health care. But it should be the same, he said. And third, conduct the analysis in a tiered approach in order to make it cost-effective.

In the literature, risk–benefit analysis sometimes shows up in disguise, for example, as risk ranking (e.g., WHO, 2015b), which Verhagen said is typically used for microbiological contamination, or as a risk–risk comparison. As an example of the latter, he mentioned a 2004 RIVM report on the public health burden of food safety versus an unhealthy diet (e.g., eating too many calories, eating the wrong types of foods), where it was found that unsafe foods contribute only about 1 percent to the public health burden (van Kreijl et al., 2004). Knowing this, in Verhagen's opinion, the best approach to increasing public health is to focus on the effect of unhealthy diets, rather than on the effect of unsafe foods. However, again, he repeated that the scientist's role is to offer the science. It is up to governmental policy makers to decide which risk to take on.

Improving Risk–Benefit Assessment

A couple of very recent developments in EFSA could contribute to improving risk–benefit assessment in the future, Verhagen opined. He mentioned a recently published report on biological relevance and weight of the evidence, specifically on the identification of effects that truly contribute to the toxicologist-defined adverse effects (EFSA, 2017b). Verhagen explained that sometimes a plethora of information is available, with not all studies pointing in the same direction. This does not mean that if there is one study that points in a different direction than another 999 studies, that one study should receive the same weight as the others. According to Verhagen, this same weight of evidence approach as described in EFSA

(2017b) can also be used to identify those effects that truly contribute to nutritionist-defined beneficial effects.

In addition to EFSA (2017b), EFSA was nearing completion of its uncertainty guidance at the time of this workshop.[4] Verhagen recalled a couple of recent developments in EFSA where clarity around uncertainty contributed to a better understanding of the message. He opined that consideration of uncertainty would be helpful in the setting of dietary reference values.

Finally, he mentioned what he considered one of the most important EFSA publications in the last 15 years: its scientific report on its PROMETHEUS (Promoting Methods for Evidence Use in Scientific Assessments) approach (EFSA, 2015). When conducting a risk–benefit assessment, the first step is to design a path, or process, he explained. The PROMETHEUS approach is a way to design this path such that after an assessment has been completed, the outcome would be essentially similar if another team of scientists were to run the same assessment at a later point. The approach leads to "good and robust science," he said.

In closing, Verhagen encouraged use of risk–benefit assessment in the future setting of dietary reference values.

DISCUSSION

Following Verhagen's presentation, he, Wells, and Lau participated in a discussion with the audience. This section summarizes that discussion.

Risk–Benefit of an Unhealthy Diet Versus Food Contamination

Peter Clifton asked about the balance between an unhealthy diet, which potentially has a very large effect, and food contamination, which potentially has a small effect. However, while the effect of food contamination is potentially small, it is also immediate and observable. "The person cannot escape it," he said, creating "quite a bit of burden" that can be "actually very serious." In contrast, even though recommendations may suggest that people change their unhealthy diets, the actual translation into action and the benefit resulting from this translation is much smaller in reality than it could be potentially.

Verhagen agreed that, in fact, the public health burden of food safety issues, particularly those related to microbiology, can be acute. However, based on calculations that served as the basis for the van Kreijl et al. (2004) report that he had mentioned, most of these infections last 1 or 2 days,

[4] The final version of this guidance was published while this proceedings was being prepared; it can be viewed at https://www.efsa.europa.eu/en/efsajournal/pub/5123 (accessed April 25, 2018).

possibly a week, then they are over, so the overall public health burden is relatively low. But there are other calculations, he acknowledged, where food contaminants contribute to lifelong effects, namely cancer. Rather than focusing on individual acute effects, he encouraged taking a population-based approach when balancing the different types of outcomes.

Dietary Reference Values: Considering Additional Health Benefits, Not Just Acute Effects of Deficiencies

James Ntambi commented on the additional beneficial health effects of increasing nutrient intake and wondered if there is any particular nutrient recommendation that has actually yielded a beneficial effect on a global scale. Verhagen responded by, first, clarifying that his interpretation of Ntambi's comment was that there may be additional health benefits to take into consideration when setting nutrient reference values, that is, benefits beyond simply the overcoming of deficiencies. Verhagen recalled that when he first became active in this field, dietary reference values were focused mostly on acute effects, such as scurvy for vitamin C. But gradually, over time, the focus shifted more toward subclinical chemical effects. Most recently, several dietary reference value studies have also begun to consider additional public health effects. He cited potassium as an example.

The Use of RCTs in Nutrition Studies

Regarding the hierarchies of evidence presented by Wells, with RCTs at the top (also, see the summary of MacFarlane's presentation in Chapter 3), Caryl Nowson commented on the fact that RCTs were designed for drug trials. When RCTs are used for nutrition trials, the doses tend to be higher because supplements are being used. For example, she has run calcium trials where participants were administered not 300 milligrams, but 1,000 milligrams. Plus, according to Nowson, none of the very few long-term trials of dietary patterns that have been run have been blinded. She asked Wells to comment on the use of RCTs for nutrition studies.

Wells agreed that RCTs are geared toward drugs, as well as devices and sometimes programs. In his opinion, one of the Achilles' heels of RCTs is the precise, pristine way they move forward, particularly efficacy trials, such as the use of a high dose of calcium in a particular population. An effectiveness trial, in contrast, would be "more real world," he said, and would apply more broadly across the population. However, even then, because a study population is never exactly the same as the target population, generalizability will always be a problem.

Lau disagreed with the notion that RCTs are not appropriate for nutrition studies. If they are well conducted, they are just as appropriate and could be very useful, in his opinion. "However," he said, "the interpretation of the results is more problematic because a lot of information is not collected."

Evidence for Risk

Patrick Stover questioned the standard of evidence for a requirement, or benefit, versus an upper level or risk. He mentioned the very well-established evidence for the role of folic acid in neural tube defect prevention. In contrast, many authoritative bodies have concluded that there is no definitive risk of colorectal cancer, although the data indicate concern and that there should be a research agenda to establish whether or not there is a risk. "How should that bar be different for risk?" he asked.

Lau replied that, when evidence is summarized, there is always uncertainty around the estimates. This uncertainty provides guidance for how strong a recommendation should be, he said. It is not just the magnitude of effect, but also the confidence interval, representing uncertainty, that should be part of decision making. The outcomes of interest and how outcomes are weighted also matter, he added.

Verhagen remarked that, in Europe, they have taken a grading approach to assessing health claims on food products. He described it as a simple, three-option approach: either a claim is substantiated by the evidence, a claim is not substantiated by the evidence, or there is insufficient evidence. Members of the European Commission have decided to accept only those health claims fully substantiated by the evidence. He mentioned the weight-of-evidence approach that he had described during his presentation, as well as the PROMETHEUS approach, as additional useful approaches to evaluating evidence.

Systematic Review Depository

Mary L'Abbé remarked that there are two approaches to applying inclusion/exclusion criteria in a systematic review. One could accept all studies initially and then conduct the quality assessment later in the process, or one could enter into review only those studies with certain qualities. She asked the speakers to comment on these different approaches.

Lau responded that, in an ideal world with unlimited resources, "you would do everything." He suggested starting with the most comprehensive, broadest review. But he also acknowledged that, because scientists live, he said, "in the real world," there are time and resource constraints. Evidence mapping can provide a sense of the scope of work that a review will require before actually extracting data. If the work appears too great, then one can constrain the review or modify the protocols. He emphasized that systematic reviews are not static and that the act of systematic review is an iterative process.

Wells agreed with Lau, adding that even if one were to do a number of different analyses, one would still have what economists call a "base case." One can start with that base case and examine different aspects of it. Additionally, he mentioned something called a "living systematic review," which he noted was a relatively new concept. Although when the Cochrane reviews began, they were intended to be updated every so often, unfortunately, Wells said, they have not been. But with the living systematic review, there is a process in place for updating the information and any recommendations that may come out of it. He mentioned a series of papers on the living systematic review that were recently published by *Journal of Clinical Epidemiology*.

Lau added that use of the SRDR will also allow for continuous updating, as well as global collaboration. He emphasized the labor intensive nature of systematic review. "If the world wants to collaborate in this effort, it becomes much easier and faster," he said.

Ruth Charrondiere agreed that the SRDR is a good step in a very good direction in terms of saving time and funds, as well as making systematic reviews more harmonized. However, she opined that one's use, or interpretation, of a systematic review depends on one's predefined view. For example, people who expected a decrease often question the results of a study that indicate an increase (or vice versa). They will wonder if the study contains a bias of some sort (e.g., if there are questions about the quality of a biomarker used to assess food consumption) or is an outlier and therefore cannot be true.

There are multiple ways to interpret results across many studies, Lau replied. For example, a sensitivity analysis could be conducted and that information made available in the results of the review. "It does not need to be a single view," he said, referring to the interpretation of results. Wells recalled some of the approximately 700-page systematic reviews that he has been involved with that have included sensitivity analyses as well as various subgroup analyses. Agreeing with Lau, he said, "Very rarely do we actually analyze it in one direction."

6

Contextual Factors: Host, Diet/ Environment, and Health Status

OVERVIEW

In session 3, moderated by Suzanne Murphy and John Muyonga, six speakers representing a wide geographic range discussed contextual factors related to host genetics and physiology, diet and environment, and health status. This chapter summarizes their presentations and the discussion that followed, with major points highlighted here and in Box 6-1.

To start the session, Patrick Stover stated that a number of physiological processes can be modified in ways that change what a nutrient requirement may or may not be. Genetics is one of these modifiers. He showed evidence illustrating that although the strongest evidence for a diet-related gene remains for the lactase gene and its evolution to allow lactose tolerance, proof-of-concept evidence exists for several other diet-related genes. But the real question, he said, is whether genetic variation in diet-related genes matters in terms of nutrient requirements. According to Stover, most genes that have an elevated effect on nutrient requirements are also high-risk factors for miscarriage, with most conceptions not proceeding to birth and, thus, naturally being selected out. He explained how variation in a common folate-related variant is a rare example of a diet-related gene that does have an effect. In 2015, the World Health Organization (WHO) used this knowledge to develop new guidelines for red blood cell folate concentrations for women of reproductive age.

Not only is variation the norm for human physiology, Anura Kurpad continued, but it is also heritable. In his opinion, the estimated average requirement (EAR) and tolerable upper intake level (UL) are not the only

BOX 6-1
Overview of Points Presented by Individual Speakers

- Genetics is one of several modifiers that can change physiological processes in ways that affect nutrient requirements. Although the strongest evidence for a diet-related gene remains for the lactase gene and its evolution to allow for lactose tolerance, there is proof-of-concept evidence for several other diet-related genes (Stover).
- Because baseline measurements of habitual intake, nutrient status, and body composition are so critically important in randomized controlled trials for nutrient requirements, it is essential that subjects be "adapted" before collecting these measurements. There can be economic consequences to setting inaccurate intake requirements as a result of not having properly adapted subjects before studying them (Kurpad).
- Infections can impair nutrient metabolism and, consequently, nutrient requirements in several ways. Two sets of nutrient intake recommendations could be considered: one for developed countries, the other for developing countries with allowance for infections (Adu-Afarwuah).
- Among other physiological changes with age, by 70 years of age, people have lost, on average, 40 percent of muscle mass and strength. Likewise with bone mass. It is important not just for physiological and metabolic responses to nutrient intakes, but also functional (e.g., risk of falls) and chronic disease outcomes (Nowson).
- There are many host-condition, dietary, and environmental factors that can affect bioavailability, thereby changing physiological and dietary requirements. More exploration of the Food and Agriculture Organization/World Health Organization Global Individual Food consumption data Tool platform as a tool for estimating bioavailability in a harmonized manner that allows for cross-country comparisons is needed (Gibson).
- Variation in bioavailability data among countries across Southeast Asia reflects the complexity of diet in Asian countries. It is not the values themselves that need to be harmonized, rather the approaches used to estimate these values. Each country still uses its own methods, despite a 2005 harmonization report that addressed how to estimate bioavailability (Fahmida).

two nutrient intake reference values that need to be measured. Variability is another. You cannot just "grab" study participants "off the road" and enroll them in randomized controlled trials (RCTs) for nutrient requirements, he said. Because baseline measurements of habitual intake, nutrient status, and body composition are so critically important, subjects need to be "normalized" before measuring these values. According to Kurpad, the consequences of not adapting subjects before studying them in an RCT can have economic consequences (e.g., if subjects are eating higher amounts of a nutrient when enrolled, their intake requirements will appear to be higher than they would be otherwise). In closing, among other reflections, Kurpad wondered if the EAR should be philosophically reconsidered with respect to what is "necessary" versus "sufficient." He pointed out that, currently, the EAR for protein, for example, is the minimum, not optimal, intake that assures balancing intake against daily losses.

The next two speakers focused on health status and its effect on nutrient intake requirements. In his overview on the role of infections, Seth Adu-Afarwuah emphasized that despite massive reductions over the past 15 years in infectious diseases in children under 5 years of age, such diseases still account for a high percentage of child mortality worldwide. He listed four ways that infections can impair nutrient metabolism and, consequently, nutrient requirements: (1) decreased food intake, (2) impaired nutrient absorption, or reabsorption, (3) loss of body nutrients (i.e., wastage), and (4) uptake, diversion, or sequestration of body nutrients. He used examples from the literature to illustrate each. "One of the hallmarks of infection is the breakdown or loss of muscle protein," Adu-Afarwuah said, in reference to the third mechanism. Data from multiple studies have all shown associations between infection and loss of nitrogen or protein. In conclusion, Adu-Afarwuah suggested considering two sets of recommendations: one for developed countries, the other for developing countries with allowance for infections.

Caryl Nowson continued the discussion on health status, but in the context of aging. Among other physiological changes with age, by 70 years of age, people have lost, on average, 40 percent of muscle mass and strength, which has a major effect on their quality of life. Likewise, bone loss with age follows a similar trend. Nowson emphasized the importance of not just physiological and metabolic responses to nutrient intakes, but also functional (e.g., risk of falls, ability to maintain activities of daily living) and chronic disease outcomes. For example, while both calcium and vitamin D have biochemical indices related to nutrient deficiency, both also have functional outcomes (e.g., fracture risk). Among other challenges in setting nutrient reference values (NRVs) for older people, Nowson questioned the extent to which functional outcomes overlap with chronic disease outcomes in this population and how NRVs for highly interrelated nutrients, like vitamin D and calcium, should be developed and communicated.

Next, Rosalind Gibson provided an overview of bioavailability. She emphasized that if host conditions, diet, or environment do not affect bioavailability, then the physiological and dietary requirements will be the same. Dietary factors known to influence bioavailability include chemical form, nature of the dietary matrix, effects of other food components (e.g., certain organic components inhibit, while others enhance), and pretreatment of food (e.g., blending, fermentation). Among the several types of methods used in the past to estimate nutrient bioavailability, the most accurate are isotopic methods based on whole diets, not single meals, according to Gibson. She discussed two types of potential tools to estimate bioavailability in a harmonized manner and allow for cross-country comparisons, The first tools would be based on food supply data from either the United Nations' Food and Agriculture Organization (FAO) food balance sheets or the FAO/WHO Global Environment Monitoring System (GEMS) cluster diet database. The second set of tools would be based on food consumption data, namely the FAO/WHO Global Individual Food consumption data Tool (GIFT) platform (FAO/WHO, 2017). She called for more exploration of the GIFT platform in particular.

Continuing the focus on bioavailability, Umi Fahmida discussed estimates of bioavailability in Southeast Asian countries that were derived using the same tools described by Gibson. She commented on the variation in iron bioavailability data obtained from isotope studies for different types of diets across India, Myanmar, and Thailand (ranging from 2–20 percent) and how this variation reflects the complexity of diet in Asian countries. Balance sheet data on energy from animal source foods show the same variation. For example, animal source foods provide 6.6 percent of energy in the Indonesia diet, compared to 21.5 percent in Brunei Darussalam. Similarly, food consumption data reveal variation in dietary intake not just among countries, but even within countries and also among life-stage groups. Fahmida shared conclusions from a 2005 report (on harmonizing recommended dietary allowances [RDAs] across Southeast Asia) regarding when and how to estimate bioavailability for what she described as "typical problem nutrients" in Southeast Asia, that is, calcium, iron, and zinc. Today, Fahmida said, despite these efforts, each country still has its own way of estimating bioavailabilities. She emphasized that it is not the values themselves that need to be harmonized, rather approaches for estimating these values.

THE ROLE OF THE HOST: GENETIC VARIATION[1]

To start the session, Patrick Stover provided a survey of the biological premise and evidence for the role that genetic variation plays in nutrient requirements. He noted that he would be essentially updating information that he had presented at the initial harmonization meeting in Florence, Italy, in 2005.

Dietary requirements are complex traits, he began. That is, there are a number of physiological processes that occur and that can be modified in ways that change what a requirement might or might not be. These modi-

[1] This section summarizes information presented by Patrick Stover, Ph.D., professor and director, Division of Nutritional Sciences, Cornell University, Ithaca, New York.

fiers include disease, epigenetics, the food matrix, nutrient–nutrient interactions, pharmaceuticals, toxins, the microbiome, and genetics. The question he said he would be focusing on for the remainder of his presentation was: how meaningful are these modifiers, in particular genetics, in terms of public health? He described this as a "hot area" of research. When the American Society for Nutrition set its research agenda in 2013, the number one priority on the agenda was to understand variability in responses to diet and food, with genetics being one of the contributing factors (Olhorst et al., 2013). Evidence for the role of genetics stretches back to the 1990s global initiative to sequence the human genome. The Human Genome Project (1990–2003) sought to determine what Stover called the "blueprint for all of life" (U.S. Department of Energy, 2017), allowing for a classification of components that make up cellular networks and determination of gene variants that modify how these networks function.

One of the most common sources of genetic variation, Stover said, are single nucleotide polymorphisms (SNPs). SNPs are single base pair differences. There are about 10 million of them in the human genome. According to Stover, although most SNPs are silent, SNPs can cause functional differences and can contribute to complex traits, such as susceptibility to chronic diseases, metabolism, and drug efficacy. Another type of genetic variation that is important with respect to diet and nutrition is copy number variation. Copy number variants (CNVs) are common variations in gene copy numbers that encode for particular proteins. They result from a duplication event, with each event increasing the amount of protein available to carry out a particular metabolic or other cell function. Like SNPs, CNVs can have functional consequences and can contribute to complex traits, including metabolism and drug resistance.

Diet and Evolution

Dietary components have been a powerful force in the evolution of all species, Stover continued (Leonard, 2002). The food that is available to a species can select for changes in the enrichment of DNA primary sequences within a population, he explained. Food can also program the genome and change gene expression. Moreover, in humans, not only have dietary components throughout evolution contributed to today's genomes, but today's human genomes, in turn, code for food tolerances and intolerances, dietary requirements, and susceptibility to metabolic disease. Where you see increased rates of diet-induced metabolic disease or associated metabolic disease, Stover said, you also often find related genome adaptions to a past environment. In its new environment, those adaptive genes are now disease alleles.

Two events need to happen for nutrition-related genetic variation to arise, Stover explained. First, there needs to be a random mutation. Then, that mutation has to expand in a population either because it confers some sort of advantage to an individual (i.e., natural selection) or because of genetic drift. According to Stover, it is now known, through computational methods, that factors related to immunity to pathogens, diet, and environmental change have been the most powerful drivers of genetic variation that determine whether an individual survives or not. These computational methods help to identify where in the genome past mutation events have wiped out preexisting variation, that is, where a new mutation that offers some sort of selective advantage has suddenly emerged and replaced all the other existent variation in the population.

According to Stover, based on what has been seen thus far computationally, the most powerful selection for a diet-related gene has been for the lactose tolerance gene (Itan et al., 2010; the lactose tolerance gene is also known as the lactose persistence gene). Expression of this gene allows humans to use lactose as a food source even as adults. The heat maps shown in Figure 6-1 illustrate a close geographic correlation between genotype and phenotype, which Stover interpreted as proof of principle that a genetic change enabled lactose to be used as a food source and that the change expanded in certain populations because it offered a selective advantage. While it is not clear if evolution of this gene was diet induced or food safety induced (i.e., with milk serving as a source of sterile liquid), "nonetheless," he said, "this is the best example we have."

Also using computational methodology, Fan et al. (2016) examined genomes around the globe and looked for local genetic adaptations that have enabled humans to live in certain areas. Among other findings, they reported that an amylase CNV that enables humans to digest starch was selected in one area, while gene variants that confer the ability to metabolize high-fat diets were selected in another area. The amylase CMV is interesting, in Stover's opinion, because it correlates well with cultures that have a history of agriculture and reliance on starchy foods for their calories. In contrast, populations that have historically been hunter-gatherers do not have as many copies of the gene.

Other diet-related genes that have similarly displayed computational signatures of selective pressure include genes for ethanol metabolism, iron homeostasis, some of the taste receptors, calcium transporters, and protein metabolism (Stover, 2007). Stover found it interesting that selection for the calcium transporter gene occurred after selection for the lactose tolerance gene, that is, that the lactose tolerance gene allowed for consumption of milk first, followed by subsequent selection for a different gene involved in calcium transport.

While all of these findings are interesting for population geneticists, the "real" question, Stover emphasized, is whether genetic variation in

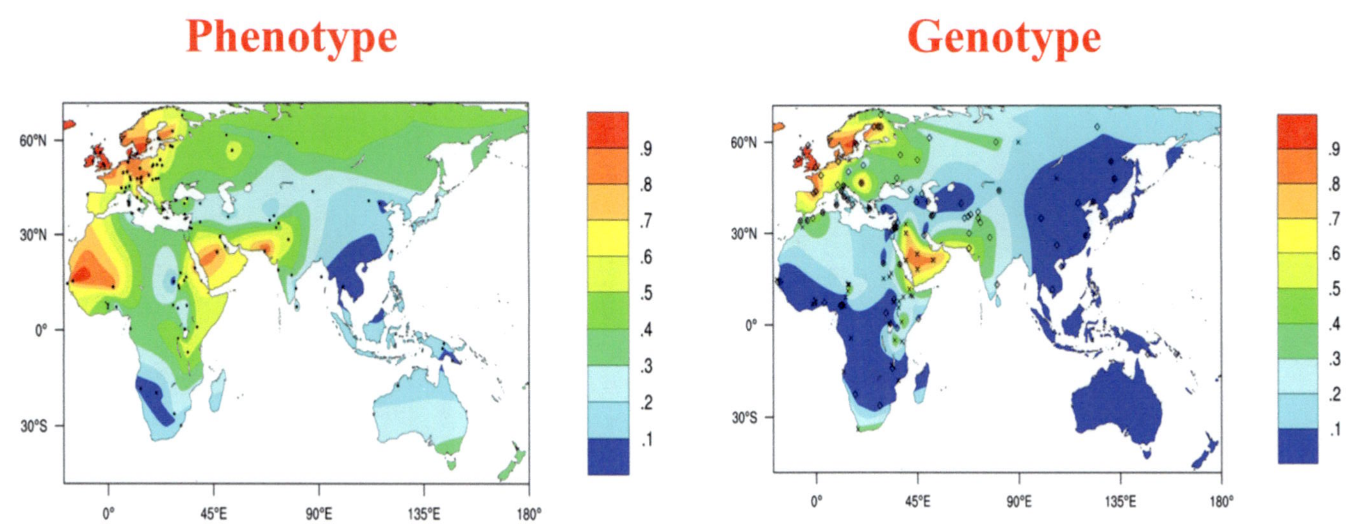

Interpolated map of Old World LP phenotype frequencies. Dots represent collection locations. Colours and colour key show the frequencies of the LP phenotype estimated by surface interpolation.

Predicted Old World LP phenotype frequencies based on LP-associated allele frequencies. LP frequency prediction assumes *Hardy-Weinberg* equilibrium and dominance. Crosses represent collection locations where all 4 currently known LP-associated alleles were genotyped, and diamonds represent collection locations where the only data on the -13,910 C>T allele is available. Colour key shows the predicted LP phenotype frequencies estimated by surface interpolation.

FIGURE 6-1 Maps of lactose tolerance phenotype frequencies ("Phenotype") and predicted lactose tolerance phenotype frequencies based on lactose tolerance-associated allele frequencies ("Genotype").
NOTE: LP = lactase persistence.
SOURCES: Presented by Patrick Stover, HMD Workshop, Rome, Italy, September 21, 2017 (Itan et al., 2010, modified with permission from BioMed Central).

diet-related genes matters in terms of nutrient requirements. The basis of personal nutrition, at least when it was first envisioned, was that genetic variation would have a highly penetrant effect on nutrient requirements. "In fact," Stover said, "that has not [been] borne out in any of the data." Only a couple of examples to date have shown an effect, because, according to Stover, gene variants with a marked effect on nutrient requirements also, by and large, are high-risk factors for miscarriage (Stover, 2007). He explained that embryos with mutations for specific nutrient requirements that cannot be met by the mother will not develop. Most do not implant, and many spontaneously abort. Thus, many of these mutations are naturally selected out during gestation. Polymorphisms in folate-encoding genes, described below, are a rare exception.

A Diet-Related Polymorphism with Policy Implications: Variation in Folate Requirement

Folate-encoding genes have many polymorphisms that can increase the risk for neural tube defects, homocysteine-related health outcomes, drug efficacy, and probably also folate requirements, Stover continued. For example, the MTHFR gene, a gene that metabolizes folate, has a common variant at base pair 677, with about 80 percent of the alleles at this position being C, coding alanine (Ala), and the other 20 percent being T and coding valine (Val). This difference has a large effect on metabolism and folate requirements, with both benefits and risks, Stover said. Individuals with the T allele have a low folate status and, thus, a higher folate requirement. They are at risk for spina bifida and, because of their higher folate requirement, miscarriage. However, if they survive gestation, they have one of the lowest rates of colon cancer known if they maintain adequate folate status (Ma et al., 1999). According to Stover, this finding has been validated in several studies. Individuals without the T allele lose that genetic advantage for cancer prevention if they become folate deficient.

The frequency of the T allele varies among populations (from 0 percent in Africans to 30 percent in Mexicans), which has implications for harmonization for nutrient standards, Stover stated, if the differences in requirements attributable to this genetic change are meaningful. Data from a large-scale study of a nonfortified Norwegian population (Fredriksen et al., 2007) showed a 32 percent difference in homocysteine (a functional indicator of folate status) and a 30 percent difference in folate status between MTHFR 677TT and 677CC homozygotes. The question is: does this difference affect nutrient requirements?

The answer is yes, he said, pointing to results of a 2008 study published in the *Journal of Nutrition*, where Solis et al. (2008) showed that folate intake at the current RDA level was inadequate for Mexican American men with the MTHFR 677TT genotype. The men were put on a controlled diet with the RDA for folate, which is 400 micrograms of dietary folate equivalents per day. Over time, homocysteine levels (again, a functional marker of folate status) among TT homozygotes went up markedly, while homocysteine levels among CC homozygotes remained the same. Stover interpreted these results to mean that, clearly, individuals have different folate requirements because of this polymorphism. "But again," he said, "this is a rare example."

In 2015, WHO used this knowledge about folate gene polymorphisms to develop new guidelines for red blood cell (RBC) folate concentrations for women of reproductive age (WHO, 2015a). This was in response to countries approaching WHO and asking about levels to which they should fortify their food supply to prevent neural tube defects. Stover explained how WHO broke the question down by deciding not to focus on either folic acid intake or neural tube defect risk, because of the errors associated with both of those measurements, but on the connection between the two: RBC folate concentration (see Figure 6-2). RBC folate concentration can be measured very well, Stover said. Then, from that measurement, one can work either backward (to folic acid intake) or forward (to neural tube defect risk). Additionally, WHO examined the effect of MTHFR status,

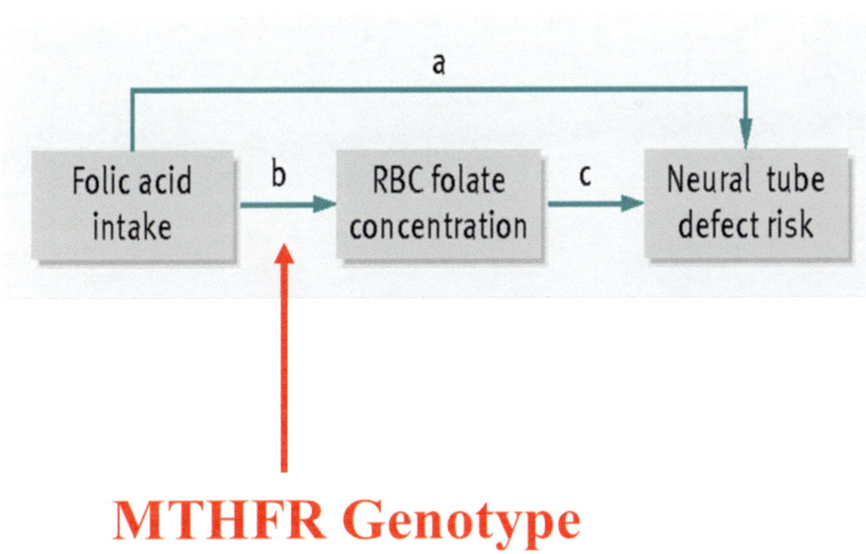

FIGURE 6-2 The Bayesian model used by WHO (2015a) to develop its new guidelines for red blood cell (RBC) folate concentrations for women of reproductive age.
SOURCES: Presented by Patrick Stover, HMD Workshop, Rome, Italy, September 21, 2017 (Crider et al., 2014, with permission from BMJ Publishing Group, Ltd.).

since it was known to be a modifier of both folate status and neural tube defect risk.

More specifically, Stover explained, using data from China, first, they ran a genotype model whose output was estimates of MTHFR genotype frequencies; then they entered that output, along with data on folic acid intake, into a concentration model whose output was estimated RBC folate concentrations; finally, they entered that output into a risk model whose output was the association between RBC folate concentration and neural tube defect risk. Through iterations of this, they computed a dose–response curve of estimated neural tube risk (per 10,000 births) as a function of RBC folate concentration (see Figure 6-3). "The beauty of this," Stover remarked, was that there were RBC clinical data from Ireland showing folate levels in all women who had a child with a neural tube defect (Daly et al., 1995). Although the generalizability of the Ireland study was unknown, nonetheless, as shown in Figure 6-3, those data overlaid very nicely with WHO's dose–response data from China.

Based on this work, WHO (2015a) was able to recommend levels of RBC folate that are needed to prevent, or reduce the risk of, neural tube defects. Countries can then decide on their own how they want to reach that level, if that is their goal, Stover explained.

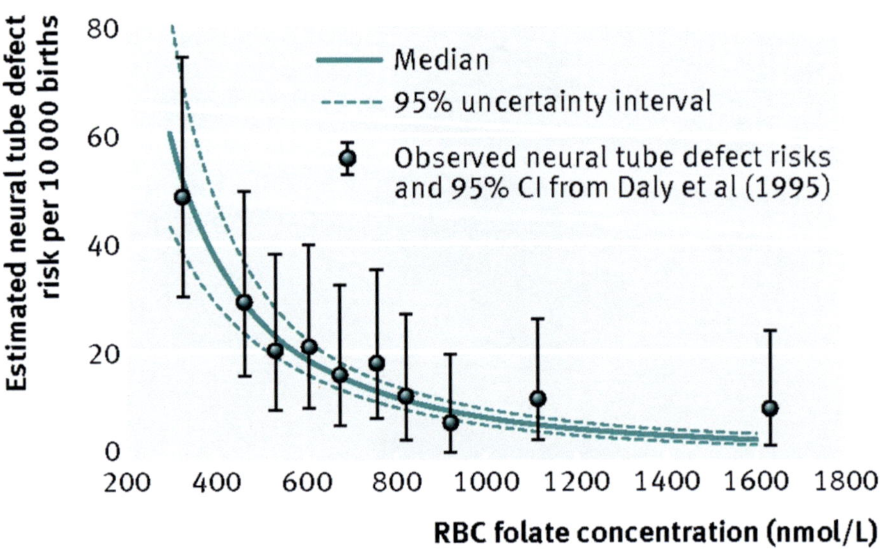

FIGURE 6-3 Dose–response curve computed from the Bayesian model used by WHO (2015a), overlaid with clinical data from Daly et al. (1995).
NOTE: CI = confidence interval; RBC = red blood cell.
SOURCES: Presented by Patrick Stover, HMD Workshop, Rome, Italy, September 21, 2017 (Crider et al., 2014, with permission from BMJ Publishing Group, Ltd.).

In closing, Stover repeated, "These examples are very rare," as they should be, based on the biological premise that genetic variants that change nutritional requirements in a way that cannot met by the mother are not going to survive. "But certainly," he said, "when they are present, like the MTHFR genotype, we have to account for them when establishing Dietary Reference Intakes."

THE ROLE OF THE HOST: PHYSIOLOGY ADAPTATION[2]

There is this idea out there, Anura Kurpad began, that physiology is the same everywhere in the world. "I'm here to tell you it's probably not," he said. According to Kurpad, it was Adolphe Quetelet, who came up with the body mass index (BMI), did so based on his belief that any variation observed was really measurement error and that a mean value described a population very well. In contrast, Charles Darwin, Francis Galton, and others viewed variation as real biology (i.e., not measurement error). Not only was variation real, but it was heritable, in their view. In Kurpad's opinion, in addition to the nutrient intake values (NIVs) mentioned by King earlier in the day as the two that really need to be measured—average nutrient requirement (ANR) and upper nutrient level (UNL)—there should be a third: variability. "I think it is very important to measure it," he said, and not just impute it or assume it. The challenge is there are different types of factors that contribute to physiological variability (i.e., interindividual variation, intraindividual variation, measurement error), all of which need to be measured.

"Normalizing" or Adapting Subjects Before Studying Nutrient Requirements

Because of this physiological variation, Kurpad said, "I think it is extremely difficult to fulfill the requirements of a clinical drug RCT for nutrients." You cannot start a nutrient requirement RCT, he said, by "getting someone off the street" and giving them doses of the nutrient under consideration. He emphasized the critical importance of the baseline measurement and the need to "normalize" study participants, or adapt them to what they normally, or habitually, eat before measuring their baseline. In addition to habitual intake, their nutrient status and body composition need to be considered as well. Too often this is not done, he said.

As an example of what he meant by adaptation, he described some of his past work with Vernon Young on the leucine requirement. They fed

[2] This section summarizes information presented by Anura Kurpad, M.D., Ph.D., professor of physiology and nutrition, St. John's Medical College, Bangalore, India.

people different levels of leucine and adapted them to those levels of intake for 7 days. Only after being adapted were subjects' leucine oxidation levels measured in the fed versus fast states. Kurpad and Young found that swings in amino acid oxidation increased the more amino acids one habitually ate. "Now, that is my point," he said, that is, that a person entering a study [on lysine requirement] at one level of an amino acid intake would react very differently at baseline than someone entering the study at a different level. Thus, people need to be adapted to whatever level the investigators decide is "normal."

Regarding the length of time needed for adaptation, Quevedo et al. (1994) showed that, when subjects are switched from a high protein intake (approximately 292 mgN/kg/d) to a medium protein intake (approximately 125 mgN/kg/d), it took about a week before the subjects' urinary nitrogen (N) excretion reached what was considered an acceptable steady state; this would be the point at which their baseline measurement for a subsequent dose in an RCT could be determined. In other work, with essential amino acids, Kurpad and colleagues had to adapt subjects for 7 to 21 days to demonstrate that a 7-day adaptation period was enough. There are consequences of not adapting subjects before they are studied, Kurpad continued. If subjects were eating high amounts of the nutrient to be studied, then their measured requirements will be higher than usual.

Another consequence of not adapting subjects is that if subjects entering a study have a larger distribution of the EAR, that is, if subjects are very variable, with some subjects eating very low amounts of the nutrient to be studied, and others eat large amounts, this will affect the estimated RDA (as opposed to the EAR), since this is determined from the distribution of measured requirements. Kurpad remarked that he has seen data from China indicating a lysine RDA that was double what he and his colleagues had determined. He explained that in the nutrition requirements world, a coefficient of variation (CV) of 10–15 percent is considered to be a reasonable CV for an EAR distribution. But, again, in studies where investigators are just "taking people off the road," without adapting them, he has seen CVs as high as 40 percent. "I think this is where we need to be clear," he said, and "harmonize all these different methods."

The Problem of Scaling

For Kurpad, in addition to the need to normalize, or adapt, subjects before studying nutrient requirements, scaling poses another challenge. He explained that requirements typically are scaled to body weight and not what he considers the "really important" components, like fat free mass. The WHO equation for basal metabolic rate (BMR), for example, is based on weight, sex, and age. However, like every prediction equation, Kurpad said, the BMR equation is dependent on the population from which the equation came. In its case, it was young army recruits from Italy who dominated the first BMR database. As a result, because those young, muscular men probably had higher than usual BMRs, the equation derived to predict BMR predicts a higher than expected BMR. The use of this same equation in India, Malaysia, or Singapore, for example, always overestimates BMR, and there are several publications that have pointed this out, according to Kurpad. In and of itself, this overestimation is not a lot. It is about 5–10 percent. But there are consequences of that overestimation, he cautioned, as the error propagates down to total energy expenditure.

A Fallacy of the Factorial Method

One would expect increased physical activity to be correlated with increased energy expenditure, based on the factorial model, Kurpad continued. However, this was not the case when Pontzer et al. (2016) collected physical activity data and measured energy expenditure in several countries worldwide. The relationship between physical activity and energy expenditure was more constrained, and energy expenditure did not increase as expected with increased physical activity. Kurpad explained that this is because there is a behavioral response that occurs when people increase their level of physical activity. In a study of semimanual laborers in India, to his surprise, he and colleagues found that the laborers actually had very low total energy expenditures. They would go to work, he said, and then come home in the evening and "sit around doing nothing, because this is the way their culture was." This meant that their work activity was nullified by extremely low leisure activity. He encouraged more thinking about the factorial method and its use for measuring requirements in children. Currently, it is the only method available, he said, but it has its fallacies.

Closing Thoughts

In closing, Kurpad repeated his concern about what "normal" is. If one is to set up a harmonized RCT and enter into the study only subjects with a baseline that has been carefully considered with respect to what normal is, the question becomes, what is normal? Again, he lamented not knowing what a unified standard of the "normal" might be, but that it depends on geography, poverty, culture, and habits. Additionally, he emphasized the importance of scaling to body composition, not weight, as illustrated by the overestimation of BMR among nonmuscular Indians (i.e., when using a BMR equation that was formulated based on data from muscular army recruits).

Kurpad also emphasized the importance of functional endpoints when setting nutrient requirements. Currently, most of these requirements are based on more readily measurable endpoints, typically physiological or biochemical losses from the body.

Finally, regarding target intake, the focus is always on the "average requirement," he said. But is the EAR an average, or is it a minimum? In fact, he said, it is the minimum intake that assures a balance with daily nutrient losses. He opined that people do not want to be told the minimum they should eat, but what is optimal for their functional health.

THE ROLE OF HEALTH STATUS: INFECTION[3]

Seth Adu-Afarwuah began by emphasizing variation in the incidence of infectious diseases between developing and developed countries. Despite massive reductions in the incidence of infectious diseases in the last two decades, infections are still common in many places worldwide. For example, in 2015, 16 percent of all deaths of children under the age of 5 years was attributable to pneumonia, with most of these deaths occurring in developing countries in the tropics (i.e., Africa, Southeast Asia, South Asia, and the Pacific). Other infectious diseases, such as diarrhea, malaria, and tuberculosis, show the same pattern, Adu-Afarwuah stated, rarely occurring in developed countries. For example, typhoid fever occurs in South Asia at a rate 10 times that in North America; and the prevalence of *Helicobacter pylori* infection is nearly 90 percent in Nigeria, compared to 9 percent in Switzerland.

Infections affect nutrient metabolism and, subsequently, nutrient requirements in four ways: (1) decreased food intake; (2) impaired nutrient absorption or reabsorption; (3) absolute or direct losses of body nutrients (i.e., wastage); and (4) uptake, diversion, and sequestration of body nutrients (Bresnahan and Tanumihardjo, 2014). Adu-Afarwuah went on to describe examples from the literature illustrating each of these mechanisms, with a focus on vitamin A and protein.

Decreased Food Intake

Adu-Afarwuah described several studies showing that infectious diseases affect nutrient requirements by decreasing food intake, beginning with a study of children in Guatemala, ages 15–60 months, who either had or did not have selected common symptoms (Martorell et al., 1980). The authors reported that children who had symptoms had a 20 percent decrease in energy intakes and an 18 percent decrease in protein intakes. Similar findings have been reported from Kenya, where children with mea-

[3] This section summarizes information presented by Seth Adu-Afarwuah, Ph.D., senior lecturer, Department of Nutrition and Food Science, University of Ghana, Legon, Ghana.

sles had a 75 percent reduction in energy consumption (Duggan and Milner, 1986). Evidence from Peru shows the same: infants with diarrhea or fever had a 5–6 percent reduction in total energy consumption or a 30 percent reduction in non-breastmilk energy intake (Brown et al., 1990). Similarly, among Bangladeshi preschool children, cholera and rotavirus infection have been shown to reduce nitrogen and fat consumption (Molla et al., 1982). As a final example, in Zambia, children with malaria demonstrated reduced energy, carbohydrate, and vitamin A consumption (Bresnahan et al., 2014).

Impaired Nutrient Absorption or Reabsorption

There are several mechanisms by which infections can impair nutrient absorption or reabsorption, Adu-Afarwuah continued. Inflammatory lesions can affect, or even damage, the proper functioning of the intestinal mucosa or cells; parasite load or size, if sufficiently severe, can affect absorptive mechanisms; interference from treatment (e.g., antibiotics) can also affect nutrient metabolism and, therefore, nutrient requirements; and, lastly, alterations in the transport system of the intestinal mucosa can affect blood flow and, consequently, nutritional requirements.

Again, Adu-Afarwuah described several studies from the literature demonstrating, in this case, that infectious diseases affect nutrient requirements by impairing nutrient absorption or reabsorption, beginning with a study of preschool children in Nigeria where the excretion of iron-labeled iron dextran, an indicator of protein loss, was higher in children with acute measles (Dossetor and Whittle, 1975). When the measles subsided, protein loss was relatively low. In the same study, lower xylose concentration in the blood, an indication of reduced absorption, reversed after the measles subsided, suggesting that the infection had impaired absorption, Adu-Afarwuah explained. In Bangladesh, preschool children with cholera and rotavirus infection absorbed less than half of nitrogen and less than half of fat; when the illnesses were over, absorption rates for both nitrogen and fat increased (Molla et al., 1982). In a study in the United States, the excretion of nitrogenous compounds, amino acids, and proteins was high in children (ages 3–9 months) with diarrhea, compared to those with no diarrhea (Ghadimi et al., 1973). As a final example, in India, preschool children with diarrhea absorbed and retained less vitamin A, compared to those with no diarrhea (Reddy et al., 1986).

Absolute Loss of Body Nutrients

Infections' effects on nutrient requirements are different than the type of loss observed during simple starvation or as a result of decreased energy consumption, Adu-Afarwuah clarified. One of the hallmarks of infection is the breakdown or loss of muscle protein and other tissues. These depletions provide a supply of amino acids to make up for the fact that, during infections, the amount of protein needed typically exceeds what is provided in the diet. Additionally, urinary loss of protein and vitamin A may occur during infections because of fever-induced damage to renal tubules. As evidence for this loss of protein, Adu-Afarwuah cited a study of people who were infected with the sandfly virus; individuals with sandfly fever symptoms excreted higher levels of nitrogenous compounds, compared to those who were not infected by the virus (Beisel et al., 1972).

Regarding the amount of protein lost during an infection, there is not much evidence, Adu-Afarwuah added, plus it is old evidence, but values between 2.5 and 3.5 grams (g) of protein per kilogram (kg) of muscle have been reported (Kocher, 1914; MacCallum, 1910). Scrimshaw (1977) reported 0.6 g protein/kg of muscle for patients with acute infection and 0.9 g protein/kg of muscle during diarrhea. According to Adu-Afarwuah, anywhere from about 0.6 or 0.9 up to 3.5 g protein/kg of muscle may be lost during an infection.

Additional examples from the literature of the absolute loss of body nutrients during infection include a study on vitamin A, where adults with pneumonia or sepsis excreted more vitamin A than a control group (Stephensen et al. 1994). In the same study, those with fever excreted more than those without fever, and individuals who were sicker excreted more than those who were not as sick. "So the excretion depends on the severity and the duration of infection," Adu-Afarwuah interpreted. In another study, children (ages 6 to 36 months) with diarrhea excreted more urinary retinol over the course of 3 days after admission to a hospital, compared to children without diarrhea (Alvarez et al., 1995). Additionally, among those with diarrhea, those with fever excreted more, compared to children without fever. Thus, again, Adu-Afarwuah explained, both infection and the presence of fever cause excretion. In yet another study, 59 percent of preschool children hospitalized for shigella experienced urinary retinol loss, with 8 percent losing more than 0.1 micromole per day (Mitra et al., 1998). Children with more severe disease excreted more vitamin A, and those with fever excreted more than those without fever.

As a final example, he mentioned a study in Brazil, where children were administered high-dose vitamin A, then, 1 month later, their liver vitamin A levels were assessed (Campos et al., 1987). At the 1-month mark, none of the children had a low liver vitamin A level. But soon after, there was a chicken pox outbreak such that, when their liver vitamin A levels were reassessed at 4 months, 10 percent of those infected had inadequate stores of vitamin A in their livers. At 6 months, 74 percent of children infected with chickenpox had inadequate liver stores, compared to only 10 percent in those who were not infected. Again, Adu-Afarwuah said, the point here is that "infection takes away a lot of the nutrient stores."

Uptake, Diversion, and Sequestration of Various Body Nutrients

Infections cause the uptake, diversion, and sequestration of various body nutrients because of the many different increased nutrient requirements needed as the body fights an infection, Adu-Afarwuah explained. For example, proteins may be needed for the production of positive acute phase proteins or the synthesis and function of phagocytic cells and immunoglobulins. Or, amino acids may be needed for energy, if the body's ability to use fat and carbohydrates is impaired in the course of infection.

As an example of evidence from the literature for this mechanism, Adu-Afarwuah cited a study of volunteers who were infected with shigella (Bostian et al., 1976). Those who developed typhoid fever showed increased synthesis of plasma proteins, whereas those who did not develop fever showed no change in plasma protein synthesis.

Implications for Harmonization

Current nutrient recommendations do not make any provision for infections. According to Adu-Afarwuah, this is partly because of the lack or scarcity of data when these recommendations were made. But additionally, arguments have been made for not making any such provision. As Adu-Afarwuah explained, it has been argued that the metabolic responses that occur with infections are purposeful adaptive mechanisms. Anorexia, for example, may be the body's way of protecting itself. It has also been argued that efficiency of the use of nutrients, which is typically very high during infection, is sufficient to allow for the repletion of nutrients during that time. Still another argument is that the focus should be on combating infections, not providing more nutrients. Finally, it has been argued that there is a "safe level of intake" that offsets the increased requirements associated with infection.

On the other hand, it has been argued that nutrient requirements should be increased when there are infections. Adu-Afarwauh explained that this argument is supported, or may be supported, by the fact that, if an individual is at borderline nutrition status, then increased nutrition could help to fight off the infection. Moreover, in this case, after the infection has subsided, one's nutrient requirements would be even higher, as the infection would have depleted body nutrients stores to a large extent. Or, he continued to explain, if a person has a marginal intake before infection, then returning to the same marginal intake after the infection has subsided would mean a longer recovery period, during which time it would make sense to increase an individual's requirements. Or, in situations where infections are frequent, increasing requirements would provide rapid repletion before the "next" disease episode. Additionally, it is known that when protein and energy intakes are increased during or immediately after an infection, this can ameliorate the negative effect of the infection.

In conclusion, Adu-Afarwuah stated that it seems, or one might argue, that the nutrient requirements for developing countries may be different than those of developed countries owing to differences in the prevalence of infection. In addition to a systematic review of the evidence, he suggested consideration of two sets of recommendations: one for developed countries, the other for developing countries that take into account the effect of infections.

THE ROLE OF HEALTH STATUS: AGING[4]

Echoing Kurpad's questioning what "normal" is, Caryl Nowson asked, "What is a normal aged person? What is expected of normal aging? What is sufficient, and what is necessary for this age group?" Her approach to looking at aging was informed by work she did with Peter Clifton while developing the framework for the NRV review in Australia (Australian Government Department of Health, 2015) (a summary of Clifton's presentation is provided in Chapter 3). When thinking about the role of aging, she always thinks about the difference between prevention of deficiency and prevention of chronic disease. It is much harder to separate these two among older adults. If the decision is made to look at endpoints for deficiency, then those endpoints need to be decided, as do the physiological and biochemical indices along that trajectory. On the other hand, if the decision is made to look at chronic disease prevention, then biomarkers need to be identified that are associated with those disease outcomes. Additionally, known interactions between nutrients also need to be accounted for, as does the population intake of relevant foods.

Physiological Changes with Age: What Is Normal Aging?

"Unfortunately," Nowson said, "we all get old, and things deteriorate." Our kidneys are not working as well, our heart is not working as well, and by the age of 70 years, on average, people have lost 40 percent of their muscle mass and strength (Janssen et al., 2000). Muscle loss, or sarcopenia, significantly affects quality of life because it requires a greater effort to move. People don't want to get out of their chairs, Nowson said. It is much easier to stay sitting. This reduced physical activity, in turn, leads to yet more muscle loss and becomes what she described as a "vicious cycle." Bone loss with age shows a similar trend, although some races are protected

[4] This section summarizes information presented by Caryl Nowson, Ph.D., professor of nutrition and aging, Deakin University, Victoria, Australia.

from bone loss to some degree, because they have higher bone mass initially, so although they decline, they don't fall into the osteopenia range (Seeman, 2003). The amount and rate of bone lost from different bones in the body varies, resulting in increased risk of fracture at specific sites such as the hip and spine. Nowson wondered whether, in an ideal world, no muscle loss or no bone loss is even achievable. "It is making me think," she said, "where are we trying to get to in terms of aging?"

Not only does deterioration happen, but the older population is a diverse mix with diverse needs. There are the well-fit elderly at one end of the range, the frail at the other end. Approximately 80 percent of adults over the age of 65 have high blood pressure, 50 percent of women over the age of 80 have a vertebral fracture, and 10 to 30 percent of adults over the age of 60 have atrophic gastritis. Based on self-reported health data, two out of three people over 65 years of age have multiple health conditions (CDC, 2013; National Center for Health Statistics, 2016). "So are we really saying that we are not going to do NRVs for those two out of three people?" she asked, in reference to the notion that NRVs are only for healthy people.

In addition to this variation in health, a whole range of lifestyle factors influence nutrient requirements in the older population, Nowson continued. For example, with respect to activity level, a sedentary lifestyle is associated with higher body fat. Obesity, in turn, is associated with low levels of circulating vitamin D. Resistance training in particular has been shown to increase muscle mass and bone density. Among adults with a mean age of 90 years, Fiatarone et al. (1994) found that 8 weeks of resistance training increased muscle strength by 180 percent and muscle size by 11 percent. "So they can do it, if you really push them," Nowson said, but "how many people are actually going to do that?" In another study, resistance training combined with higher protein intake led to an increase in muscle mass and strength (Houston et al., 2008). But again, Nowson asked, how many people are going to do this? These findings raise the question: when making nutrient recommendations, how should this type of exercise, as well as other lifestyle factors, be taken into account?

Other lifestyle factors that can affect nutrient requirements in the older population include smoking, which can have lifelong effects on bone density; high alcohol intake throughout life; industrialization, with the highest hip fracture rates in North Europe and the United States and the lowest in Latin America and Africa; and latitude, with a north–south gradient in fractures, which Nowson noted is perhaps related, to some degree, with vitamin D and cultural practices (i.e., covering up in the sun), as well as the effects of clouds and pollution on ultraviolet (UV) exposure (Bow et al., 2012; Dhanwal et al., 2011; Ensrud, 2013).

Protein: Functional Outcomes

Nowson emphasized the importance of looking at protein in terms of functional outcomes, not just physiological and metabolic responses (Campbell et al., 1994, 2001; Castaneda et al., 1995). Protein-related functional outcomes include falls, fractures, and activities of daily living. These functional outcomes are also affected by interrelationships with other nutrients, like vitamin D and dietary calcium; medications; and the home environment. Nowson commented on the need to dissect these out when making recommendations and the fact that there remain unanswered questions around how to do that. She cited a 2013 FAO report on protein quality, where it was argued that future efforts should be directed toward looking at long-term health outcomes, including age-related function, bone strength, and chronic diseases (FAO, 2013).

There is no one specific physiological index of protein deficiency, although there are a number of indices that can provide an indication of the protein status of the body. Body weight reflects total body mass, including muscle which is related to both energy and protein intake. Dual-energy X-ray absorptiometry (DEXA) measurements provide measurements of body composition, including the amount of muscle. There are also indices of muscle strength such as hand grip. Although all of these are affected by inadequate intake of dietary protein, they are also affected by a range of other factors, including energy intake, vitamin status (e.g., vitamin D), and level of physical activity. Biochemical indices are not very reliable for older people, according to Nowson. For example, nitrogen balance has not been shown to be a robust marker, because older people adapt to a lower protein intake by breaking down some of their muscle mass, although, she noted, new methods may assist with that (Castaneda et al., 1995).

Calcium and Vitamin D: Functional Outcomes

With calcium and vitamin D, again, as with protein, one could measure physiological or biochemical indices of deficiency. But again, with respect to biochemical indices, serum calcium levels are of no use, Nowson remarked, and there are questions about the use of calcium balance studies given the unrealistic expectation that there will be no bone loss at 80 or 90 years of age, likewise, with physiological indices, such as bone density. She asked, "Do we really expect to have the bone density of a 30-year-old [at 80 or 90 years of age]?"

While some experts have called for a target level of serum 25(OH)D (i.e., above 80 nmol/L) for normal functioning, in Nowson's opinion, there is no good evidence for this (Forsythe et al., 2012). However, she noted there is a clear increased risk of rickets at 25(OH)D levels less than 30 nmol/L and an apparent risk of osteoporosis at levels less than 50 nmol/L. While vitamin D status is related to calcium absorption at relatively low dietary calcium intakes, she said, "Again, it doesn't give you the whole picture." Several aging-related conditions, including reduction in body weight, muscle mass, and physical activity, negatively affect total body calcium, with subsequent reductions in bone mineral density resulting in structural defects. Other nutrients can also affect calcium balance and, consequently, bone mineral density and structure. For example, insufficient protein can adversely affect calcium absorption, while a higher sodium diet can increase calcium excretion.

Functional outcomes related to calcium and vitamin D deficiency include osteoporosis, fractures, and falls, all of which occur, Nowson noted, with low bone density (Kenney and Prestwood, 2000). Overlaying all of this, vitamin D deficiency is associated with osteomalacia (inadequate calcification of the bones), as measured by bone biopsy, as well as with a reduction in muscle strength. Although many vitamin D supplementation trials have reported a reduction in falls and fractures, these reductions occur primarily before there is any effect on the bone, so they may be muscle related.

Bones at old age, she explained, are dependent on genetic makeup and the accumulation of what has happened throughout life, including the amount of bone built up during early life. Much of the prevention of osteoporosis has been an effort to increase bone density during childhood, as doing so reduces risk of falling into the "fracture zone" at an older age, Nowson explained. While women lose bone more rapidly during menopause, everyone experiences bone loss with age, which raises the question for Nowson, "How much can we actually have an impact on that?"

Global Patterns in Calcium and Vitamin D

Although the global patterns of calcium supply and deficiency risks reported in Kumssa et al. (2015) show where the greatest deficiency risks are, including in Africa and India, these patterns do not correlate with fracture outcomes, Nowson continued.

The global distribution of low vitamin D status among elders, as reported in Palacios and Gonzalez (2014), shows no "frank deficiencies" (i.e., less than 30 nmol/L) and low levels (19 percent) of moderate deficiency (below 49 nmol/L) in Canada. This is probably because of mandatory fortification, Nowson noted. In the United States, the frank deficiency rate is 5 percent, the moderate deficiency rate 34 percent. Like Canada, the United States has higher levels of fortification in its food supply. Rates in Australia are 7 percent frank deficiency and 17 percent moderate deficiency. Some of the highest rates of deficiency are in Morocco (52 percent frank deficiency, 85 percent moderate deficiency), India (62 percent frank deficiency, 91 percent moderate, 98 percent mild [less than 75 nmol/L]), and the Middle East.

Australia has been conducting campaigns around safe sun exposure, Nowson said, but the campaigns are complicated because two out of three Australians will be diagnosed with skin cancer before the age of 70. So there is a risk to recommending sun exposure. Plus, skin-produced vitamin D lasts in the circulation two to three times longer than a supplement of vitamin D, and evidence is emerging that high serum levels may have some adverse effects (Haddad et al., 1993; Holick, 2012; Wacker and Holick, 2013). In addition to sun exposure and vitamin D supplementation, a range of other factors can affect vitamin D status, including age, ethnicity, skin color (people with darker skin need to be out in the sun up to six times as long for UV light to trigger the conversion of inactive vitamin D to active vitamin D), physical activity, skin cancer risk (people who have had skin cancer avoid sunlight), food supply fortification, and dietary intake of calcium.

Possible Challenges in Setting NRVs for Older People

To close, Nowson summarized the challenges in setting NRVs for older people in the form of questions:

- What is a "healthy" older person?
- Currently, NRVs are set for older people between 50 and 70 years of age and for people over the age of 70 years. Is that what we should be using? Or, is functional age, however that is defined, a better categorization?
- What is a functional deficiency outcome? What is a chronic disease outcome? How much do these outcomes overlap in this older population?
- What is the gap between the population intake to prevent a deficiency and the population intake to prevent a chronic disease?
- How much weight should be given to high-dose supplement trials, particularly in populations where nutrient intake is traditionally low? Most of these trials, Nowson said, involve high-dose supplements. There are very few lower-dose trials. She was unaware of any trials that have persisted long enough to examine, for example, the effect on bone outcome of a "good" diet, but with less calcium or other nutrients.
- How should NRVs for nutrients that are highly interrelated, like calcium and vitamin D, be described and communicated?

THE ROLE OF DIET AND ENVIRONMENT IN SETTING NUTRIENT BIOAVAILABILITY FACTORS FOR ESTIMATING DIETARY REQUIREMENTS[5]

Rosalind Gibson began her presentation by defining bioavailability: To convert physiological requirements into dietary requirements, an adjustment is often needed to take into account factors that affect the proportion of the ingested nutrient that is absorbed and used through normal metabolic pathways (Hurrell et al., 2004). Bioavailability can be influenced by several factors, including diet and environment—which is the focus of Gibson's talk—but also genetic variation and host health. However, if host conditions, diet, or environment do not affect bioavailability, then the physiological and dietary requirements will be the same, she emphasized. Gibson defined bioefficacy (e.g., as currently applied to provitamin A) as the efficiency with which ingested nutrients are absorbed and converted to an active form.

Factors That Affect Bioavailability

Currently, according to Gibson, there are sufficient data to quantitatively assess the effect of dietary factors on the bioavailability or bioefficacy for only certain nutrients, namely protein, the trace elements iron and zinc, and certain vitamins. These vitamins include folate, particularly the difference between food folate and synthetic folic acid (i.e., in supplements and fortificants); the difference between food vitamin B12 and crystalline B12; and preformed retinol versus the provitamin A carotenoids. For other nutrients, such as selenium and niacin, there are not enough quantitative data to adjust for bioavailability, noted Gibson.

Dietary factors known to influence either bioavailability or bioefficacy include chemical form, nature of the dietary matrix, effects of other food components, and pretreatment of food. Gibson described each of these in detail. Regarding chemical form, it is known that the bioavailability of iron, zinc, folate, and carotenoids is influenced by their chemical form. Regarding the nature of the dietary matrix, it is known that folate and carotenoids are involved.

With respect to the effects of other food components, there are certain organic food components known to inhibit and others known to enhance the bioavailability of certain micronutrients. According to Gibson, these include the following:

---

[5] This section summarizes information presented by Rosalind Gibson, Ph.D., M.S.P.H., professor emerita, Department of Human Nutrition, University of Otago, Dunedin, New Zealand.

- Phytate, polyphenols, and oxalates, all of which inhibit the bioavailability of certain minerals (see the paragraph at the end of this section for Gibson's discussion of the inhibitory effect of phytate on zinc);
- Pectin and lignin, both components of dietary fiber that are known to inhibit fat-soluble vitamins, carotenoids, and protein;
- Organic components, such as organic acids, which are known to enhance the bioavailability of iron and zinc;
- Vitamin C, which is known to enhance the bioavailability of iron;
- Animal protein, which is known to enhance the bioavailability of iron, zinc, and copper; and
- Fat, which is known to enhance the fat-soluble vitamins and carotenoids.

Additionally, it is known that interactions between micronutrients tend to occur only with high doses of supplements and without food.

Regarding the pretreatment of food, Gibson continued, it is known that preparation, processing, and cooking can all influence the bioavailability of certain micronutrients. Specifically, it is known that the milling of unrefined cereals reduces the phytate and mineral content; soaking can actually reduce the content of water-soluble phytate and simultaneously reduce some water-soluble minerals and B vitamins; blending can enhance the bioavailability of carotenoids and folates; and germination or fermentation can reduce the phytate content, as a result of enzyme-induced hydrolysis, and simultaneously increase the bioavailability of iron, zinc, and calcium.

Regarding phytate, Gibson explained that recent stable isotope work of Michael Hambidge and coworkers has demonstrated that the inhibiting effect of phytate on zinc absorption is much greater than previously estimated (Rosado et al., 2009). Their data on total absorbed zinc as a function of total dietary zinc at six different levels of phytate have been used by the European Food Safety Authority (EFSA) to generate the dietary zinc requirements for adult males and females at four different levels of phytate, ranging from 300 to 1,200 milligrams per day (EFSA NDA, 2014). In addition, Gibson noted, it is known that people in low-income countries, whose diets are mainly plant based, often have phytate intakes that exceed 1,000 milligrams, meaning that their estimated zinc requirements are probably very high.

Methods Used to Estimate Bioavailability

Several methods have been used in the past to estimate nutrient bioavailability: animal models; in vitro methods; in vivo methods, including isotopic methods; and changes in biomarkers or functional outcomes. Of these, Gibson said, the most accurate are the isotopic methods, which have been used to assess the bioavailability of iron, zinc, calcium, folate, and vitamin A. It is now known, she added, that isotope studies are most accurate if they are done on whole-day diets, not single meals. The earlier studies on single meals have been shown to have exaggerated the effect of absorption modifiers.

As an example of the use of isotopic methods to estimate bioavailability, Gibson cited WHO/FAO (2004) data showing that a diet with very high meat in two main meals daily and high ascorbic acid has a 27.5 percent iron availability, compared to a diet with negligible meat or fish, high phytate, high tannin, and low ascorbic acid, which has a 5.5 percent iron bioavailability. These calculations were based on a woman weighing 55 kg and with no iron stores and assuming an intake of 15 mg of iron daily.

Additionally, for some nutrients, isotopic methods have been used in combination with mathematical models to develop bioavailability algorithms and classify diets into high, medium, or low bioavailability. As an example, she cited WHO and FAO's use of isotopic data, along with other data on food consumption patterns, to develop algorithms for both iron and zinc. Diets for each nutrient are classified into three groups: high, moderate, and low bioavailability.

For iron, the low bioavailability diet is 5 percent bioavailability (simple, monotonous diet of cereals, roots, and/or tubers; negligible amounts of meat, poultry, and fish, or ascorbic-acid rich foods); the moderate bioavailability diet is 10 percent bioavailability (diets mainly of cereals, roots, and/or tubers; minimal amounts of meat, poultry, fish, and ascorbic acid); and the high bioavailability diet is 15 percent bioavailability (diversified diet with generous amounts of meat, poultry, fish, and/or with high amounts of ascorbic acid).

For zinc, the three groups are also based on the phytate:zinc molar ratio. The low bioavailability diet has an estimated 15 percent bioavailability, with a phytate:zinc ratio greater than 15 (cereal based with greater than 50 percent energy from unrefined cereals or legumes; negligible animal protein); the moderate bioavailability diet has an estimated 30 percent bioavailability, with a phytate:zinc ratio between 5 and 15 (not based on unrefined cereal grains or high-extraction rate [> 90 percent] flours); and the high bioavailability diet, with its estimated 50 percent bioavailability, has a phytate:zinc ratio less than 5 (low in cereal fiber; animal foods major protein source). More recently, Gibson continued, the International Zinc Nutrition Collaborative Group (IZiNCG) developed an algorithm for zinc that is based on more up-to-date whole-day diets only and which includes only two diets, one a mixed/refined vegetarian diet with a phytate:zinc ratio between 4 and 18, the other an unrefined cereal-based diet with a phytate:zinc ratio greater than 18.

New Tools for Estimating Bioavailability Across Countries

Next, Gibson considered several potential tools that might be used to estimate bioavailability across countries in a harmonized manner that allows for cross-country comparisons. These tools make use of available food supply data, either from FAO food balance sheets or the WHO/FAO GEMS/Food cluster diet database, or food consumption data from the FAO/WHO GIFT platform (FAO/WHO, 2017).

The FAO food balance sheets, Gibson explained, are available for 210 countries. They provide per capita values for the supply of 95 food commodities expressed in grams per day and for energy, protein, and fat. These data can also be used for other nutrients, as has been done for zinc and phytate. As an example of data generated from the FAO food balance sheets, she referred to data from Wessells and Brown (2012) on mean daily per capita phytate:zinc ratios and fractional zinc absorption (as a percentage from the available food supply). The data are available by both region and country. The methods and assumptions that were used to generate the data are described in Wessells et al. (2012). The fractional zinc absorption percentages were calculated using the updated trivariate model in Miller et al. (2007).

The WHO/FAO GEMS/Food cluster diet data are from 183 countries. The data have been standardized into 13 cluster diets, providing, again, a means for characterizing data across countries. Finally, the FAO/WHO GIFT platform, in Gibson's opinion, would be the preferred data to use because it is based on individual dietary intakes by life-stage group. It provides mean daily intakes of standardized food groups in grams per day, as well as nutrients, antinutrients, and food sources of nutrients.

She described several different indicators that could be used to estimate bioavailability, or bioefficacy, by country and life-stage group, when GIFT data become available. These include food-based indicators, either selected food groups (g/day or g/kg body weight/day) or selected foods (e.g., red meat, liver, maize, rice, orange-yellow fruits and vegetables, green leafy vegetables), both of which could be used to estimate iron, zinc, or vitamin A bioefficacy. Or, nutrient-based indicators might include: total protein, indispensable amino acids, or dietary fiber, all of which could be used to estimate the bioavailability of protein; major food and food group sources of nutrient intakes, which could be used to estimate the bioavailability of calcium or vitamin A; or the proportion of iron or zinc from fresh foods, which could be used to estimate iron and zinc bioavailability. Other potential indicators that might be calculable from GIFT data include heme iron and nonheme iron (to provide an estimate of the bioavailability of iron) and phytate:zinc molar ratios or fractional zinc absorption (to provide estimates of zinc bioavailability).

Environmental Factors

Gibson briefly discussed the one environmental factor known to have the potential to influence nutrient requirements: exposure to UV light from sunshine. Specifically, it is known that such exposure influences the extent of endogenous synthesis of vitamin D in the skin. At higher latitudes, where UV light is decreased, less vitamin D is synthesized in the skin and, thus, more is needed from the diet. She added that although there may be other environmental factors that may also influence nutrient requirements (e.g., extremes in ambient temperatures, exposure to high altitudes, exposure to pollution, pesticide exposure), there are not enough data to actually quantify particular effects.

Closing Remarks

In conclusion, first, Gibson thought it important to remember that physiological requirements must be adjusted to dietary requirements to account for bioavailability of certain nutrients. Second, she suggested that current quantitative iron algorithms may have limited use across populations, whereas the Miller trivariate model for estimating bioavailability of zinc does have that potential, particularly with the advent of the new FAO/International Network of Food Data Systems (INFOODS)/IZiNCG phytate database. Third, she encouraged exploring use of food balance sheets, GEMS, and particularly the new GIFT initiative so diets can be classified more accurately in terms of iron and zinc bioavailability in habitual diets across populations. Fourth, she mentioned that the dietary requirement for vitamin D is the only nutrient adjusted for environmental exposure (i.e., UV light) at the present time.

Additionally, she summarized some approaches to consider for harmonizing the adjustment of bioavailability across countries:

- Reach consensus on which nutrients need to be adjusted for bioavailability. Does the list need to be increased?
- Reach consensus on which isotope data need to be selected for bioavailability estimates, in view of the fact that it is now known that there is a big difference between using whole-day diets versus single meals.
- Explore the use of GIFT indicators for classifying diets as low, intermediate, or high bioavailability for iron and zinc across countries.
- Consider calculating dietary phytate:zinc molar ratios across countries using national food consumption survey data and the new phytate database; and exploring application of the Miller trivariate model for estimating fractional zinc absorption across countries.

- Explore the use of GIFT indicators on the major food sources of provitamin A carotenoids to more accurately estimate the bio-efficacy of vitamin A across countries.
- Calculate folate bioavailability by taking into account both food folate and folic acid from fortification and supplements, where relevant.

To close, Gibson emphasized that many countries now have national food consumption data available. However, in New Zealand, for example, the statisticians who analyze the data do not really understand their many potential uses. "We could be using these data much more than we have used them in the past," she concluded.

THE ROLE OF DIET ON NUTRIENT BIOAVAILABILITY: ISSUES FOR HABITUAL DIETS OF ASIAN COUNTRIES[6]

Umi Fahmida continued the discussion on bioavailability, with a focus on habitual diets in Southeast Asian countries. She noted the tools used to estimate bioavailability in the Asian region are the same as those described by Gibson, with isotopic studies being the "gold standard." As Gibson had, she also mentioned the FAO food balance sheets, which profile data from 210 countries; the WHO/FAO GEMS/Food cluster diet data from 183 countries; and National Food Consumption Survey (NFCS) intake data from the FAO/WHO GIFT platform, although not all countries are included in the GIFT platform, she noted, including Indonesia. She then went on to share some examples of bioavailability estimates from these different sources.

The Use of Isotopic Data to Estimate Bioavailability

According to Fahmida, iron absorption data obtained from isotopic studies were among the first reference data available for bioavailability in countries across South and Southeast Asia; these were the same data used by WHO/FAO (2004) to develop its algorithm for iron bioavailability. These data indicated that even within a single country, iron bioavailability can differ greatly among different types of diet. In India, for example, Narasinga Rao et al. (1983) reported iron absorption rates of 1.7–1.8 percent for a millet-based diet, 3.5–4.0 percent for a wheat-based diet, and 8.3–10.3 percent for a rice-based diet; in Myanmar, Aung-Than-Batu et

[6] This section summarizes information presented by Umi Fahmida, Ph.D., deputy director, Southeast Asian Ministers of Education Organization Regional Center for Food and Nutrition, Universitas Indonesia, Jakarta, Indonesia.

al. (1976) reported rates of 1.7 percent for a rice-based diet, 5.5 percent for rice diet plus 15 grams of fish, and 10.1 percent for a rice diet plus 40 grams of fish. In Thailand, Hallberg et al. (1974, 1977) reported rates of 1.9 percent for a rice-based diet, 4.8 percent for a rice-based diet plus 100 grams of fresh fruit; and 21.6 percent for rice diet plus 60 grams of fish. This variation reflects the complexity of the diet in Asian countries, Fahmida remarked.

Use of Food Balance Sheet Data to Estimate Bioavailability

Food balance sheet data have been used to estimate energy obtained from animal source foods across Southeast Asian countries, expressed as both total kilocalories per day and percentage energy from animal source food. For example, in Indonesia, only 6.6 percent of energy comes from animal source foods, compared to in Brunei, where 21.5 percent of energy comes from animal source foods. These same data can also provide more specific information for use in estimating bioavailability, Fahmida explained. For example, using 2005 food balance sheet data, Wessells and Brown (2012) estimated percentage of energy from animal source foods (5.8 percent in Indonesia), as well as percentage of energy of zinc from animal source foods (17.5 percent in Indonesia) and zinc fractional absorption rates (28 percent in Indonesia). What is interesting about these data, Fahmida pointed out, is that, although the percentage of zinc from animal source foods varies among countries (e.g., again, with the highest rate in Brunei, where 43 percent of zinc is obtained from animal source foods), the estimated fractional zinc absorption rates are quite similar across countries, for example, 23.5 percent in Brunei, compared to the 28 percent in Indonesia. Fahmida explained that this is because other food components also affect the bioavailability estimate (i.e., the phytate:zinc molar ratio).

Use of Food Consumption Data to Estimate Bioavailability

The problem with food balance sheet data are that they pertain to *available* food, not actually consumed food, Fahmida continued her explanation. The best estimates for actual intake come from NFCS data. For example, using NFCS data from South Korea and China, respectively, Kwun and Kwon (2000) and Ma et al. (2007) reported information on the bioavailability of iron, zinc, and calcium not just in terms of total intake (10.1 mg zinc per day in South Korea, 10.6 in China; 15.2 mg iron per day in South Korea, 21.2 in China; and 426.5 mg calcium per day in South Korea, 338.1 in China), but also in terms of phytate:mineral molar ratio and the extent to which this molar ratio was above a desirable cutoff. Additionally, both research teams broke down their estimates by life-stage group and by urban versus rural setting. This breakdown, Fahmida commented, illustrates how different bioavailability estimates can be derived within a single country.

As an example of how NFCS data have been used in Indonesia, Fahmida shared data on estimates of the percentage of pregnant women consuming cellular animal protein (96.0 percent), vitamin C–containing foods (24.2 percent), orange and yellow fruits and vegetables (20.4 percent), and green leafy vegetables (96.2 percent), as well as frequency of consumption per week and median portion size. These data can be used to estimate bioavailability of habitual diet for specific target groups (e.g., pregnant women). She noted that these data can also be broken down by area.

Harmonization in Southeast Asia

In 2005, a report was issued following a series of meetings in Southeast Asia on the harmonization of RDAs (ILSI, 2005). Fahmida shared some conclusions from that report that she said typify the challenge of estimating bioavailability in Southeast Asia. For example, with calcium, it was decided that dietary calcium content was of greater importance than bioavailability, especially because the intake of dairy products in Asia is often very low. Additionally, the report concluded that calcium was poorly absorbed from foods rich in oxalic acid (e.g., spinach, sweet potatoes, rhubarb, beans) or phytic acid (e.g., unleavened bread, raw beans, seeds, nuts, grains, soy isolates); and that data on calcium absorption from specific foods were limited because the effects of absorption modifiers had not been quantified. Given these considerations, the committee decided that it would not consider bioavailability when setting calcium dietary requirements in the region.

For iron, again, Fahmida repeated that diets in Southeast Asia are too complex to estimate bioavailability for all habitual diets using isotope techniques. Although the committee concluded that the development of algorithms was an attractive alternative to isotopic studies, they also concluded that more work was needed to quantify the effects of various components in Asian diets affecting iron bioavailability. For example, while the new phytate database by FAO/INFOODS/IZiNCG will permit estimates of phytate:iron molar ratios from NFCS data, in fact, Fahmida said, tannin is the most important inhibitor of iron. But there is no consensus yet on the analytical methods needed to estimate tannin. In the meantime, the 2005 committee concluded that it is reasonable to assume, based on available scientific data, that iron bioavailability in Southeast Asia ranges from 5 to 10 percent. To account for this range, the ILSI (2005) committee recommended RDAs for iron based on three different levels of bioavailability: 5, 7.5, and 10 percent.

For zinc bioavailability, the committee deferred to the use of food balance sheet data to estimate fractional zinc absorption and also recommended using the FAO/INFOODS/IZiNCG phytate database to estimate phytate:zinc molar ratios from NFCS dietary data. Additionally, they recommended that fractional zinc absorption (as a percentage) be calculated using individual-level NFCS data, using the updated Miller equation (Miller et al., 2007).

Fahmida remarked that, today, each country has its own RDAs, but it is not the values themselves that need to be harmonized, rather, because of the diversity of habitual diets across Southeast Asia, it is the approach to setting these values that needs to be harmonized.

In summary, Fahmida reiterated that iron bioavailability, given the complexity of the diet in Asian countries, is difficult to estimate. While there is the potential to use algorithms, the challenge is in making additional food consumption data available, for example, for tannin intakes. For zinc, while food balance sheet data allow for estimates of fractional absorbable zinc, in Fahmida's opinion, a better option would be to use NFCS data so bioavailability estimates are based on food intake, not food availability, and will allow breakdown of bioavailability estimates by specific life-stage groups. Finally, for calcium, although calcium is a problem in Asian countries, Fahmida said, data are still insufficient to quantify the effects of absorption modifiers and, thus, bioavailability is not considered when setting calcium dietary requirements in Southeast Asian countries.

DISCUSSION

Following Fahmida's presentations, she and the other five speakers in this session participated in an open discussion with the audience, summarized here.

The Globalization of Numbers Versus Methods

A question was asked about whether global harmonization is even possible, given the many factors that can influence nutrient intake values. In response, Murphy reminded workshop participants that the goal of the workshop was to consider not global harmonization of numbers, but of methods. She suggested that perhaps an outcome of this workshop would be to consider whether all of the information presented can be compiled into a procedures manual to provide guidance to regions or countries that want to set their own nutrient recommendations.

Kurpad further clarified the difference between approach and value. He said, "There is a way to be global in your approach to setting standards. You needn't get the same value." Murphy agreed with Kurpad, then said, "But I think it is easy to listen to this long list of factors and say it is just hopeless to even think about harmonizing." She repeated that the purpose of this workshop was not to discuss setting global numbers, rather global procedures for setting numbers, something that she thought is possible.

Nonetheless, the original question led to continued discussion about whether single numbers are possible. Caroline Spaaij pointed out that the United States and Canada together set single values despite variation across such a large region. She asked, "Why wouldn't it be possible to set a value even at a larger scale?" When Stover responded that he thought the political barriers were much steeper than the scientific barriers, Spaaij agreed, but still questioned why reference values are set at higher or lower levels in different countries. There are other reasons why this is the case other than differences in bioavailability, she opined. For instance, some organizations set reference values based on clinical relevancy in preventing deficiency symptoms, while others set values to be on what she called the "safe side." The clinical relevancy of the latter is less clear. She added that, at least in the reports that she has examined, most reference values are based on a few critical references repeated across reports. Yet, she said, these same references yield different values in the different reports.

Przyrembel suspected that the scarcity of good data may explain why the same references are always showing up in different reports. Gibson emphasized the importance of using an evidence-based approach and the need to provide countries with advice on how to select studies in the literature from their own countries. For instance, many people are selecting studies with bioavailability data that are based on single meals, rather than on whole-day dietary intakes. If countries were advised on how to select studies and provided criteria, in her opinion, this would really help to reduce some of the discrepancies across countries.

Kurpad questioned whether something more sinister than biology and health might be at play in setting requirements. He agreed with Spaaij that there are agendas behind the setting of requirements. In his opinion, international transparency is probably the best way to sort through this problem.

Bioconversion for Beta-Carotene

Klaus Kraemer commented on the need to address bioconversion in addition to reference values. He pointed to EFSA's scientific opinion in 2015 to stay with the WHO/FAO 1:6 retinol activity equivalent (conversion of beta-carotene to vitamin A; WHO/FAO has been using the 1:6 ratio since 1967, according to Kraemer), even though the Institute of Medicine suggested a 1:12 ratio. (As summarized in Chapter 7, Emorn Udomkesmalee also commented on the change in use of these two ratios.)

Hidden Issue: Environmental Enteropathy

Additionally, Kraemer commented on what he considered a largely hidden issue: environmental enteropathic disorder. The workshop discussion has addressed infections and specific physiological states, he reflected, but people in many developing countries, because of hygiene, water, and sanitation issues, are experiencing a situation that may lead not necessarily to diarrhea, but to a leaky gut and chronic inflammation which, in turn, significantly affects nutrient demand. "There is very little known about that," he said.

Calcium Balance in Southeast Asia

Clifton asked if calcium intake is a problem in Southeast Asia. His studies have suggested that one does not need the "Western kind of RDA" of calcium per day (e.g., 1,300 mg) to be in calcium balance and that people with intakes of 300–400 mg per day can be in balance. He wondered whether any calcium balance studies have been done in Southeast Asia. Prentice questioned why such data were even necessary, given the health and longevity of the population even at low calcium levels. Fahmida was not aware of any existing data from Southeast Asia on calcium balance, but repeated that calcium is considered a "problem" nutrient in the region with respect to intake level. Clifton remarked that it is only a problem compared to WHO suggested calcium levels, which he said, were Western based, not Asian based.

Warren Lee referred workshop participants to recent work by Connie Weaver and colleagues. Using isotopes to study absorption, they were surprised to find that Chinese immigrants in the United States required less calcium and could reach calcium balance at a lower level, compared to Caucasian subjects. This is because they have a higher absorption rate and also a lower excretion rate, Lee explained. He cited this as an example suggesting that there might be physiological differences between groups, in this case between ethnic Chinese and Caucasians. In response to Lee, Clifton suggested that baseline diet matters. Among people who drink a lot of milk and have had high calcium intakes their whole lives, their calcium absorption is switched off, essentially. In contrast, among people who do not drink milk, calcium absorption increases. Lee added that similar differences have been found between white and black Americans, with black Americans tending to have higher calcium absorption and also higher bone accretion, even though they have lower calcium intake compared to white Americans. And unlike the ethnic Chinese, he noted, black Americans were born in the United States (implying that their baseline diets are similar).

7

Breakout Discussions: Applications, Facilitating Quality, and Cost-Effectiveness

OVERVIEW

The breakout discussions in session 4, moderated by Lindsay Allen, were designed by the planning committee to encourage all workshop participants to provide input into ways to harmonize methods for setting nutrient reference values. Each breakout session addressed one of three questions (i.e., two groups per question): (1) What are the advantages of global harmonization of methodologies for developing nutrient intake recommendations, from your standpoint? (2) What additional resources and expertise would facilitate adoption of a harmonized approach in your region/country? (3) What are the likely barriers and challenges to achieving global harmonization from your standpoint? Afterward, representatives from each discussion reported back to the workshop participants on strategic points made by individual discussants. Their reports are summarized here. As is true of this report in its entirety, the opinions and ideas summarized here are those of individual workshop participants and should not be construed as consensus. Also included in this chapter are summaries of Catherine Leclercq's introduction to the breakout discussions, Allen's synthesis of the breakouts, and the open discussion that took place afterward.

SETTING THE STAGE[1]

Leclercq set the stage and provided guidance for the breakout discussions by emphasizing that addressing the three questions was not to be an academic exercise, that is, the goal was not to list advantages or barriers in a theoretical way, but rather to identify actual advantages and barriers. She urged participants not to be "good wishers," that is, not to simply respond to others by saying, for example, "oh, what a nice initiative," but to be outspoken and honest and to think about what has really been important in their own work or in the work of colleagues or other institutions. She cautioned that if actual barriers are not identified, those same barriers will still exist 10 years from now, and she urged identification of actual advantages so institutions can move in those directions.

By way of illustration, she told the story of her own "relationship" with nutrient intake recommendations, beginning when she was a Ph.D. student conducting a survey on the intake of sodium. At the end of her work on the survey, she wanted to see how well intakes in the population aligned with recommendations. At the time, she said, that was an easy comparison to make, as there was only one recommended value, the World Health Organization (WHO) population goal.

But later in her career, while serving on a committee in Italy to derive nutrient intake recommendations, she was challenged by how few resources were available. This is still true today, she remarked, as is the case with many countries. But back then they did not have the European Food Safety Authority (EFSA), only documents from the European Commission. Yet, those documents proved "so useful," she said, because they provided the committee with a regional nutrient intake recommendation that they could then adapt for their own country. She agreed with a comment from the previous day regarding the value of regional nutrient intake recommendations, especially for countries with few resources.

Later, Leclercq was involved with a nationwide survey in Italy, one that she described as quite comprehensive and with quite good quality data on food consumption for a large number of nutrients and vitamins. Those data have been published since then and used widely. However, they were unable to assess dietary adequacy (except for macronutrients). According to Leclercq, doing so would have required a dedicated Ph.D. student to study the assumptions and approach needed to estimate usual intake and other variables for each nutrient. The significance of this, she interpreted, is that even in Italy where many resources are available, they were unable to assess dietary adequacy for nutrients and minerals.

---

[1] This section summarizes information and opinions expressed by Catherine Leclercq, Ph.D., nutrition officer, Nutrition and Food Systems Division, Nutrition Division, Food and Agriculture Organization (FAO) of the United Nations, Rome, Italy.

Most recently in her professional life, Leclercq joined the United Nations' Food and Agriculture Organization (FAO) and was recruited to develop the FAO/WHO Global Individual Food consumption data Tool (GIFT).[2] She described the tool as being useful not only for developing nutrient intake recommendations, but also for using nutrient intake recommendations to assess adequacy. However, she admitted that the latter application has been a "bit slow" and has been done thus far only for vitamin A. Vitamin A was, she said, "the easy one." For the next nutrient, they will need to consider political issues, for example, whether to use old WHO values or more recent values that come from a specific institution. She explained that the tool allows users to input any nutrient recommendation, either FAO's or a user's own.

Leclercq emphasized that the focus of this workshop was *global* harmonization, that is, harmonization that serves not just EFSA, the United States, Canada, and other large countries that have many scientists and skills, but harmonization that serves the world. She pointed out that, in fact, most people live in Asia. Additionally, she encouraged workshop participants to keep in mind women and children, including pregnant women; people who are doing hard work; and people who grow old. Consider how harmonization work will cover their needs, she urged. Will it influence these people when they are eating at home? Will it influence their consumption out of the home, such as when children are at school? She predicted that the influence would be more controlled where food is being distributed (e.g., at school) or when supplements are provided.

Additionally, she encouraged stakeholders to keep in mind the intermediate end user, such as people who are developing standards for school meals. She mentioned a survey on school meal standards in 33 low-income countries that found only three countries using their own standards even though many of these countries had their own nutrient intake recommendations. The other 30 were relying on the U.S. school meal standards. She mentioned people who are involved with dietary assessments as another intermediate end user to keep in mind when thinking about harmonization.

Finally, she cautioned against developing a harmonized process that requires the same level of skills and resources currently relied on in the United States, Canada, and the European Union. She encouraged stakeholders to keep in mind countries not represented at this meeting, for example, countries in Latin America.

In closing, she encouraged stakeholders to be concrete, but also to be inspired; to think globally; and to consider end users not present at the workshop.

---

[2] Both Rosalind Gibson and Umi Fahmida discussed GIFT in their presentations, which are summarized in Chapter 6.

QUESTION 1: ADVANTAGES OF GLOBAL HARMONIZATION OF METHODOLOGIES

As reported by Amanda MacFarlane and Anura Kurpad, participants in the two breakout groups assigned to the first question described three strategic advantages of global harmonization:

- Many individuals identified a *better use of limited resources* as one of the primary advantages. Discussants described a streamlined approach that would make better use of limited resources to set nutrient reference values, one that might allow resources to be directed to nutrients that have been ignored in the past because of lack of resources, lack of evidence, or inattention to important subgroups (e.g., pregnant women, children, elderly).
- A second, related advantage identified by many discussants would be *increased country-level application* of nutrient reference values derived by harmonized methodologies, such as the development of food-based guidelines. Kurpad described use of the same resources (i.e., those made available through harmonization) as "cutting to the chase." As an example, there was some discussion in one of the groups around iodine intake levels and how countries could save time by using the U.S.-defined upper limit for iodine and applying it to local situations.
- Yet another, related advantage identified by several discussants would be *increased scientific capacity*, including expertise for particular nutrients. Kurpad described the greater pool of scientists that would be made available, one extending across regions, as a "global village," with everyone being available to everyone.

Other advantages identified by individual discussants, again, as reported by MacFarlane and Kurpad, included

- Increased transparency around setting nutrient reference values;
- Increased trust and confidence among both governments and consumers in the science that emerges from having a transparent harmonized approach and in the recommendations stemming from that science;
- Empowerment of countries and regions to set their own nutrient reference values and to implement these values to meet their needs;
- Facilitation of the global trade of staples and processed foods (e.g., through the use of similar nutrient requirements for staples and unprocessed foods or through the use of standardized labels and claims for processed foods);

- Easier identification of gaps in knowledge once a common scientific paradigm is in place, with several individuals pointing to gaps in knowledge around folate requirements as an example; and
- Opportunities for a transparent, open access systematic review repository.

Additionally, Kurpad relayed that several individuals in his group had discussed the value of a harmonized single number in addition to a harmonized process, perhaps across regions. "We're not saying that you should have one," he said, "but we're not saying that you shouldn't have one." In his opinion, a single number would help to standardize criteria for trade and food.[3]

QUESTION 2: ADDITIONAL RESOURCES AND EXPERTISE TO FACILITATE ADOPTION OF A HARMONIZED APPROACH

As reported by Umi Fahmida and Joseph Lau:

- Several individuals in both breakout sessions identified an evidence repository as the number one additional resource needed to facilitate adoption of a harmonized approach. They envisioned a repository containing a wide range of information, not just systematic reviews, but also food composition tables, food consumption data, bioavailability data, and other related data. Additionally, some discussants envisioned that, for the sake of transparency, this information repository would also include detailed documentation of processes. Others imagined a database occupying a single spot online where anyone can access it.
- Many individuals also envisioned a technical brief, or guide, with the brief containing detailed methods not only for developing nutrient recommendations, but also for adjusting recommendations to allow for differences in genetics, physiology, infection, aging, and bioavailability. Additionally, several participants also envisioned a statistical software package to support the technical brief, as well as an online or face-to-face collaborative training on use of the manual.
- Some individuals identified regional networks as an additional needed resource, with each network representing the different countries' nutritional societies.

[3] See Chapter 6 for a summary of some earlier discussion on this same issue: the difference between harmonizing processes, which was the focus of this workshop, versus harmonizing numbers.

- In addition to training users of the technical brief, some individuals suggested training on how to use the nutrient recommendations themselves. There was some concern expressed that, currently, many countries do not use nutrient intake recommendations appropriately. As with the training for the imagined technical brief, it was suggested that such a training course be made available either online, so it is easily accessible, or through collaboration.
- Finally, some discussants identified the need for a feedback mechanism to ensure that actual food intakes align with derived nutrient recommendations.

QUESTION 3: LIKELY BARRIERS AND CHALLENGES TO ACHIEVING GLOBAL HARMONIZATION

Discussants identified a multitude of barriers and challenges to achieving global harmonization, as reported by James Ntambi and Laura Martino:

- Reluctance to accept global harmonization, not only among end users, but also politically.
- Confusing terminology, with different terms being used to define the same concept and different concepts being associated with the same term, such that even very basic aspects of the discussion create obstacles. Some individuals discussed how even the term *recommendation* has multiple interpretations.
- Lack of resources, not just funding, but also scientific interest, including lack of new scientists who want to work in this area.
- Lack of data in some countries or populations, for example, the HIV/AIDS population.
- The scattering of data, including data not in the public domain
- Heterogeneity in the quality of data.
- Lack of openness, or sharing, of data, technology, and results because of legal or political constraints.
- Inherent uncertainties and lack of transparency around recommended intake values and the implicit and explicit assumptions underlying those values, which makes it difficult for a country to adopt other countries' numbers or to develop its own values. Martino commented that sometimes the population to which a value or method applies is not clear. For example, she asked, what is meant by "healthy adults"?[4]

[4] See the summary of Caryl Nowson's presentation on aging in Chapter 6 for some earlier discussion on this same issue.

- Difficult decisions about inclusion versus exclusion of evidence when setting recommendations and differences among countries and regions in how these decisions are made.
- Different endpoints among countries and regions.
- Differences in the updating of recommendations.
- The difficulty of bringing existing methodologies from different regions or countries together.
- Lack of scientific platforms in some countries, including access to information on harmonization (e.g., at meetings like this).

SYNTHESIS OF BREAKOUT DISCUSSION[5]

Lindsay Allen was asked to synthesize the breakout discussion and highlight what she interpreted as main points. This section summarizes her synthesis.

A main advantage of global harmonization is that it could generate more resources into setting nutrient intake recommendations, she began. She described three additional advantages: (1) empowerment of countries, nutrition societies, and others; (2) improved translation of information, because there would be information available on how to use the data; and (3) increased transparency around where the numbers (i.e., nutrition reference values) come from.

Critical additional resources needed to facilitate adoption of a harmonized approach include not only sources of funding, Allen continued, but also a data, or information, repository. She described the data repository as one that could contain a wide range of information, including available systematic reviews and other scientific evidence, food composition tables (which she noted are mostly online already, but could be converged), and bioavailability data. As had the discussants, she envisioned that such a repository would engender larger bodies of scientific expertise around particular nutrients.

Additionally, Allen highlighted the need for a technical brief, or methods manual, coupled with software and some form of training (e.g., online, face to face, via scientific collaboration or country nutrition societies). The manual should detail the harmonized process methodology and should include clear terminology, separate assessment methods for each nutrient, information on how to set bioavailability values, guidance on when to include or exclude data, guidance on how to set endpoints, and instructions for how to interpret the software.

---

[5] This section summarizes information and opinions presented by Lindsay Allen, Ph.D., center director, Agricultural Research Service Western Human Nutrition Research Center, U.S. Department of Agriculture, Davis, California.

Regarding challenges to harmonization, Allen emphasized the need to convince stakeholders everywhere that a harmonized approach is needed, first, by explaining why it is needed and, second, by providing examples. Other main challenges, in Allen's opinion, are variable terminology, lack of scientific platforms and resources, and questions about how readily people will actually share information nationally, regionally, or internationally.

DISCUSSION

The discussion following Allen's synthesis revolved around three main issues: the potential effect of harmonization on future research, the potential for data to be misused, and how harmonization of methods can help when data are missing.

How Will Harmonization Affect Research?

Allen wondered what harmonization would mean for nutrition research. Specifically, she asked, by having a harmonized process in place that empowers people to set their own guidelines, "Are we actually wiping out the need to do research on this?" Would it slow research in countries without resources and inhibit development of original data? Or, on the other hand, would it create interest? Hasan Hutchinson opined that an available methodology for all would stimulate research by making it easier to identify gaps and problems with implementation in particular regions. Allen responded that, while Hutchinson's prediction may be very true in countries with more resources, her concern was with countries with few resources.

The Potential for Misuse of Data

In response to the many calls for a database located in a single place and accessible to everyone, Anura Kurpad cautioned, "We live in a world of social media . . . data can be misused as well." One of his concerns was the many things that can be done in a systematic review that are not necessarily transparent, such as removing a single study, which, he said, can "ever so slightly change things around so that you get what you want." But an even bigger worry for him is that people without knowledge of the biology of what they are looking at will apply these freely available databases and methodologies and develop recommendations. He expressed uncertainty regarding how this potential for misuse could be regulated. Additionally, he cautioned that creation of a harmonized methodology must also consider the consequences, particularly in terms of medicalization.

Martino agreed that misuse is a risk, as it is with any scientific paper (i.e., people can extract data and misuse them), but she emphasized the importance of sharing information. No individual scientist, institution, or country can do this alone. "We have to be aware of the risks and address them," she said, "but not stop this process."

In fact, there are a couple of ways to address these risks with respect to systematic reviews, George Wells explained. First, at the beginning of a systematic review, protocols for the review are often published and openly available, similar to the way ClinicalTrials.gov publishes information on clinical trials.[6] Second, systematic reviews can be transparent and reproducible if information is provided in the review for a third party to reproduce the review, ensure that the original review actually followed the protocol and did not cherry-pick evidence, and verify the results of the original review.

Harmonization When Data Are Missing

In response to the many comments that had been made during the breakout discussion about lack of data, Patrick Stover pointed out that this workshop was about harmonization. He asked, "Shouldn't we be talking about, 'How do you harmonize approaches when there are no data?' What do you do? Isn't that the big question?"

Leclercq emphasized making clear that the proposed technical brief should address not only how to use primary data but also how to extrapolate from existing data and adapt those data to other countries or age groups. Especially for small countries, this section of the brief may be the most useful part, in her opinion. Ruth Charrondiere agreed that an added challenge is the large amount of missing evidence not just for some geographic areas, but also for some age groups, like infants and children.

Allen imagined that use of data would be a critical component of the manual, given that most countries do not even have access to numbers they can use as average requirements or upper levels.

[6] Guidance on accessing U.S. registered clinical trial protocols is available at https://ClinicalTrials.gov/ct2/help/for-researcher (accessed May 18, 2018).

8

Exploring Advantages, Barriers, and Challenges to Global Harmonization of Methodologies for Nutrient Intake Recommendations

OVERVIEW

In the final session, moderated by Susan Fairweather-Tait and Amanda MacFarlane, panelists shared experiences from countries that have collaborated with other countries or entities to develop nutrient intake recommendations. This chapter summarizes these presentations and discussion, with major points highlighted here and in Box 8-1.

First, Christophe Matthys provided an overview of how the EURRECA (European Micronutrient Recommendations Aligned) network has addressed a range of scientific questions and policy development issues, beginning with how to define endpoints in the determination of nutrient requirements. EURECCA's approach, he described, is based on three criteria: (1) new scientific evidence, (2) public health relevance, and (3) heterogeneity in existing recommendations (e.g., different vitamin D recommendations in neighboring countries). EURRECA's other work revolves around:

- translating physiological requirements into recommendations, particularly in the case of uncertainty;
- questions on the added value of a scientific advisory body and issues around stakeholder involvement;
- the use of nutrient recommendations in policy making; and
- involvement of consumers in dietary guideline development, with a main challenge being how to explain uncertainty.

BOX 8-1
Overview of Points Presented by Individual Speakers

- Among its other scientific and policy development work, the European Micronutrient Recommendations Aligned network (EURRECA) built an evidence pyramid for prioritizing micronutrients to review. The pyramid is based on three criteria: (1) new scientific evidence, (2) public health relevance, and (3) heterogeneity in existing recommendations (Matthys).
- A challenge to global harmonization and one that the European Food Safety Authority (EFSA) has faced in its own work will be finding experts with enough time, knowledge, and readiness to travel. Another challenge, again, one that EFSA has faced in its own work, will be finding consensus in a heterogeneous group of experts. Between-country technical conferences and better between-institution communication when setting nutrient reference values should be encouraged (Przyrembel).
- Africa has faced a range of challenges to harmonization. This includes limited capacity to handle food and nutrition issues and the scattering of information across academic institutions and interested agencies. Thus, the challenge for Africa is not only to develop a unified approach, but to build the capacity needed to do so (Ntambi).
- For decades, Norway has been collaborating with the other four Nordic countries to develop nutrition recommendations, with the most recent edition issued in 2012. The significant role of systematic reviews is this last revision. Given the enormous amount of time and work that they required, a nutrition specialty in systematic reviews is called for (Meltzer).
- The wide range of recommended protein intake across Southeast Asia, even when comparing similar age groups, reflect differences in "judgment." There is a critical need for guiding principles that the Dietary Reference Intake committees can use when there is no clear "yes or no" decision (Udomkesmalee).

Unlike EURRECA, which Hildegard Przyrembel described as a project, the European Food Safety Authority (EFSA), she emphasized, is an institution. Specifically, EFSA is an independent organization that assesses and communicates risks associated with the food chain, but it is not allowed to make recommendations in nutrition. She discussed EFSA's recent growth in response to a 2005 request from the European Commission to revise and add missing values to the 1993 dietary reference values (DRVs). In Przyrembel's opinion, the approach for setting reference values is similar in different regions of the world. The difference, she said, lies in the amount of money, personnel, knowledge, data collection, and time available. Thus, one of the challenges to harmonization, and one that EFSA has faced, is finding experts with enough time and knowledge and the readiness to travel. Another challenge, she observed, is finding consensus in a heterogeneous group of experts. But there are advantages too, she continued, such as EFSA's comprehensive databases on food consumption and composition. She encouraged between-country technical conferences and better between-institution communication when setting nutrient reference values.

James Ntambi offered insights into several challenges to harmonization across Africa:

- limited capacity to handle food and nutrition issues, including nutrient intake values (NIVs);
- diversity in foods, dietary patterns and habits, seasonal food supplies, and agricultural practices (e.g., the nutrients in plantain in one region may be very different than those in plantain in another region);
- the reality that the challenge is not only to develop a unified approach to determining NIVs, but to build the capacity needed to develop this approach both in individual countries and across Africa as a whole;
- the scattering of information among academic institutions and interested agencies; and
- questions around how to coordinate existing national and regional bodies across Africa that handle food and nutrition issues. He noted that many of these organizations have begun the process of generating NIVs, but have run out of resources.

Even though Norway is considered "one of the richest and best countries in the world," Helle Margrete Meltzer said, it cannot afford to develop guidelines on its own. It has been collaborating with the other four Nordic countries for decades, most recently on the fifth edition of nutrition recommendations (issued in 2012). The fifth edition, according to Meltzer, focuses on nutrients of particular relevance to the Nordic countries, namely vitamin D, iodine, iron, and fatty acids and fats. Of note, it was also the first revision that involved working with systematic reviews. Because working on systematic reviews was new to most of the approximately 100 nutrition experts involved with the revision, combined with the fact most of the reviewers were unpaid and working during their free time, it was, she said, a "huge undertaking." It was a slow process, one with many pitfalls (e.g., conducting systematic reviews requires knowledge about biases) and with large volumes of publications to examine. One of the "learning points" from this work, Meltzer concluded, is that, in her opinion, global harmonization will require a nutrition specialty in systematic reviews.

The final speaker of this session, Emorn Udomkesmalee called attention to the wide range of recommended protein intakes across Southeast Asia. For example, among 4- to 6-year-olds, the recommended protein intake is 35 grams per day (g/day) in Indonesia, 21–22 g/day in the Philippines (females/males), 25 g/day in Vietnam, and 16 g/day in Malaysia. Such differences across very connected countries is "why we are here," she said. In her opinion, it is not the approach to setting recommendations that is the problem, as all of these countries use similar approaches. Rather, the problem, she said, is judgment. These countries are challenged by limited expertise on local committees and major gaps in relevant data, even when setting recommendations for healthy populations. Udomkesmalee called for harmonized guiding principles that countries can follow when decisions need to be made and evidence is missing. More specifically, she called for harmonized guiding principles that address the diversity in context among countries.

EURRECA (EUROPEAN MICRONUTRIENT RECOMMENDATIONS ALIGNED)[1]

Christophe Matthys provided an overview of critical scientific questions and policy development issues addressed by the EURRECA network. Funded under the European Union Sixth Framework Programme Network of Excellence, EURRECA brought together many universities that are working on setting micronutrient recommendations. Its aim was to conduct preparatory work for EFSA, although there has been some political discussion around the relationship between EFSA and EURRECA, Matthys remarked. He noted that EURRECA is coordinated by International Life Sciences Institute (ILSI) Europe, and ILSI Europe receives part of its funding from the food industry. In his opinion, source of funding is yet another challenge to harmonization, in addition to those identified during the breakout discussion, as listed in Chapter 7.

Matthys summarized EURRECA's work as a series of five questions, beginning with how to define endpoints in the determination of requirements, taking into account public health importance, available new evidence, and priority populations. He noted that, when discussing physiological aspects, EURRECA always discusses requirements, not recommendations, as the latter are considered risk management and the former risk assessment and therefore "purely science," he said. Matthys described the scheme by Cavelaars et al. (2010) for prioritizing micronutrients to review based on three criteria: (1) new scientific evidence, (2) public health relevance, and (3) heterogeneity of recommendations. As an example of the latter, he explained that he lives in Belgium, with the Netherlands just a 1-hour, 50-kilometer drive away from his home. Yet, based on current vitamin D

[1] This section summarizes information presented by Christophe Matthys, Ph.D., assistant professor, Human Nutrition, University of Leuven, Belgium.

recommendations, he would need to increase his vitamin D intake by a factor of five if he were to go the Netherlands. He and his EURRECA colleagues, such as Cavelaars et al. (2010), searched PubMed for studies on inadequate intake and status and their association with health outcomes, focusing on randomized controlled trials since 2003. They examined studies by population group and then built a multidimensional evidence pyramid for each group. Each pyramid has four tiers, with the top tier occupied by evidence that fulfills all three criteria (i.e., new, relevant for public health, heterogeneous), the second and third tiers occupied by evidence that fulfills only two of the criteria (either new and relevant for public health or new and heterogeneous), and the bottom tier being evidence that fulfills only the "new scientific evidence" criterion. Matthys remarked that these priority pyramids allow EURRECA to divide its resources based on evidence and to move forward.

The second question EURRECA's work revolves around, Matthys continued, is how to translate requirements into recommendations, using the coefficient of variation (CV) in cases of uncertainty. Matthys described the creation by Dhonukshe-Rutten et al. (2013) of a conceptual framework to develop a projected "requirement distribution" and projected "optimal scenario" for each micronutrient. Although the projections are based mostly on dose–response curves for different health outcomes, Matthys explained that in certain situations, for example, for certain population groups, they had to rely on the factorial approach.

Because recommendations have to be "read," Matthys said, this raises the third question around which EURRECA's work revolves: What is the added value of a scientific advisory body, and how can representatives of the different stakeholders be included? He described how Timotijevic et al. (2011) looked at the way different scientific advisory committees across Europe were working and found that, in some countries, it was very clear how these committees were working, with very transparent documents and decisions and clear terms of reference about the composition of the committee and its tasks. But in other countries, it was, Matthys said, "the one who shouted the most" who decided what a reference value would be. Thus, he said, "There's really a clear need to have a specific framework." He added that the framework should also allow for consumers to rely on and understand what experts are doing.

Regarding stakeholder involvement, Matthys said that there is a clear north–south gradient in Europe, with a lot of involvement of stakeholders in the northern countries. In the south, in contrast, most food and nutrition policy decisions are made by experts and policy makers, not stakeholders. In Matthys's opinion, when thinking about stakeholder involvement, another question to consider is how to include the hard-to-reach part of the population, especially immigrants, in the development of recommendations.

The fourth question around which EURRECA's work revolves is on the use of nutrient intake recommendations in policy making. Matthys noted that EURRECA conducted an inventory of nutrient-related policy types and instruments across Europe and found a big difference among countries (Timotijevic et al., 2013).

Finally, the fifth question, involvement of consumers in dietary guideline development, with a main issue being how to explain uncertainty to a consumer, has led EURRECA to many discussions on the effect of a change in a recommendation on the population (Brown et al., 2013). For example, if the recommendation for vitamin D were to change from 2.5 to 2.6, based purely on the science, what effect will that have? How can the relevancy of that change be explained to consumers? Another issue is the selection of consumers to contribute to discussions on recommendations. In Belgium, for example, it is often the same people speaking at the food safety agency stakeholder meetings, Matthys observed.

EFSA (EUROPEAN FOOD SAFETY AUTHORITY)[2]

Hildegard Przyrembel began by emphasizing that EFSA is an institution, in contrast to EURRECA, which is a project. More specifically, EFSA, founded in 2002, is an independent scientific source of advice, information, and risk communication on risks associated with the food chain. "We are not allowed to make recommendations," Przyrembel emphasized.

EFSA's opinions and advice are formulated by the scientific committee and the scientific panels, which, in turn, are composed of external, independent experts who are recruited on the basis of an open application process. No one is admitted, Przyrembel noted, unless someone thinks that he or she has competence in some field. The balance of men and women is okay, according to Przyrembel, as is the balance among countries. She described it as a very difficult selection procedure, but one that she thinks EFSA manages well.

EFSA's work on DRVs began with a 2005 request from the European Commission to revise the existing population reference intakes from 1993 (SCF, 1993) and to add missing values for DRVs not set in 1993. As a first step, the Panel on Nutrition, Dietary Foods, and Allergies wrote a 2010 opinion on principles for deriving and applying DRVs (EFSA NDA, 2010). Przyrembel described how, based on many papers, particularly from the Institute of Medicine (IOM), but also from member states, a decision was made to define:

[2] This section summarizes information presented by Hildegard Przyrembel, M.D., Ph.D., professor and director emerita, Federal Institute for Risk Assessment, Berlin, Germany.

- average requirement (AR),
- population reference intake (PRI), which she noted was equivalent to the King and Garza (2007) NIV,
- lower threshold intake (LTI),
- adequate intake (AI) (if average requirement cannot be defined), and
- reference intake range for macronutrients (RI).

Przyrembel noted that RIs have also been defined for some micronutrients as well, when no agreement could be reached on a point value for PRI.

These values are set by working groups, with additional external experts invited when they are known to have special knowledge for a particular nutrient and with the support of EFSA scientific officers, statisticians, and the data unit (evidence management), Przyrembel explained. She noted that EFSA has grown over the last 14 years from a very small unit into what she described as a "very impressive institution."

The approach for setting reference values is similar across different regions of the world, Przyrembel remarked. She stated that this is particularly true of the AR, provided the criteria are fulfilled. In her opinion, differences in how these values are set lies in differences in the amount of money, personnel, knowledge, data collection, and time available. Based on her experience, a main challenge in this work is finding experts with enough time, knowledge, and readiness to travel. A second challenge is finding consensus in heterogeneous groups of experts with different backgrounds and varying levels of expertise in a particular field. "You learn a lot when you are on one of these scientific panels," Przyrembel said. "There is always somebody who knows something else, and perhaps better."

Regarding the advantages of "this setup," Przyrembel continued, one is that, as of about 3 years ago, protocols can now be written for literature searches and appraisals of pertinent papers to permit systematic reviews of the available evidence. In the past, Przyrembel recalled, nutrition panels relied on the collecting ability of the experts in a panel. So now, it is done on a more systematic basis, because of an increased demand for transparency and replicability of panels' assessments. The literature searches are often outsourced to external contractors.

Another advantage is the backup provided by EFSA's databases on food consumption and food composition.[3] Przyrembel described the database

[3] Przyrembel was referring to the EFSA Comprehensive European Food Consumption Database (http://www.efsa.europa.eu/en/food-consumption/comprehensive-database) (accessed June 13, 2018) and the EFSA Nutrient Composition Database (http://www.efsa.europa.eu/en/data/food-composition) (accessed April 25, 2018).

as a comprehensive one that covers all member states of the European Union and is divided by category (i.e., age, food group, type of consumption [regular and high consumption]). It allows for calculations for each category of consumer and intake of any nutrient. Also worth mentioning, in Przyrembel's opinion, is the anthropometry database for European children between the age of 0 and 18 years (van Buuren et al., 2012). EFSA's reference body weights for children to 2 years old are those of the World Health Organization (WHO) growth standard, she said, but those for older children are based on this database. She cautioned, however, that if EFSA's DRVs were to be used in other settings in other regions of the world, they would need to be adapted.

Although EFSA received some priorities for activities from the European Commission when it started this work, it was free to choose the sequence, Przyrembel recalled. Thus, it has relied on other mechanisms for setting priorities, as necessary, including systematic reviews, technical briefs, and toolkits. In addition to relying on the 2010 opinion paper on how to derive DRVs and the means needed for assessment (EFSA NDA, 2010), between-country technical conferences are also sometimes convened to find out which DRVs are universally applicable and which are not. In Przyrembel's opinion, these conferences could be held on a greater scale. She urged more conferences between institutions that set up NRVs as a way to explain differences in results.

In Przyrembel's opinion, the potential for acceptance of methodological approaches across countries exists in the European Union. Given that EFSA is a huge, well-working institution with financial and personnel resources that are so much greater than of any single member state, she wondered, "Why do member states make less use of the work which is done there?"

Moving forward, she called for mutual recognition and respect and, whenever feasible, cooperation. She suggested identifying the most urgent problems and tackling them first or selecting from available NRVs those that need population- or region-specific reassessment.

In closing, Przyrembel mentioned a recently completed DRV summary report that contains summaries of all of the opinions, but also provides information (on how the values were decided) in tabular form by age and sex (EFSA, 2017a).

AFRICA[4]

James Ntambi offered insights into the challenges to harmonization across Africa, beginning with Africa's limited capacity to handle food and

[4] This section summarizes information presented by James Ntambi, Ph.D., professor of nutritional sciences, University of Wisconsin–Madison.

nutrition issues, including NIVs. Compounding the challenge, Africa has diverse foods, dietary patterns and habits, seasonal supplies, and agricultural practices. Additionally, in contrast to developed countries, where most foods are processed, most foods consumed in Africa are natural foods, and because of regional differences in seasons and soils, this means that the composition of these natural foods may be very different. For example, the nutrients in plantain in one region may be very different than the nutrients in plantain in another region. Because of this diversity, Ntambi continued, harmonization will require not only building capacity in individual countries and across Africa as a whole, but also developing unified approaches and methods to determining NIVs. He expected that this will require use of existing well-developed, science-based methods.

He was aware of work that had been done in Uganda to determine nutrient content in some foods, such as iron in amaranth, but information on similar work on other nutrients was scattered across many academic institutions and interested agencies. He suspected that this was the case for other African countries as well. Additionally, he remarked that while there are existing national and regional bodies in Africa that were formed to handle food and nutrition issues, the question is, how can all of these bodies be coordinated and harmonized with a greater global system?

In his opinion, harmonization is possible. In fact, the process started in Uganda and East Africa and part of southern Africa, but they ran out of resources. "There is an opportunity to restart," he concluded.

NORWAY[5]

Norway is considered "one of the richest and best countries in the world," Helle Margrete Meltzer began, "but even with that starting point, we would never be able to afford to make dietary guidelines on our own." Fortunately, she said, the country has a long history of very close, good collaboration with the other four Nordic countries. Since 1980, their collaboration on nutrition recommendations has been supported by the Nordic Council of Ministers, with the fifth edition published in 2014. According to Meltzer, because resource constraints make it out of reach to fully reassess every nutrient when revising the recommendations, they put their main emphasis on those nutrients with specific issues or challenges of relevance to the Nordic countries. For instance, vitamin D, iodine, iron, and fats and fatty acids have almost always been on the agenda.

For this last edition, for the first time, they worked with systematic reviews. In the past, they relied on what Meltzer described as "knowledgeable

[5] This section summarizes information presented by Helle Margrete Meltzer, Ph.D., research director, Norwegian Institute of Public Health, Oslo, Norway.

professors." But that was back when individual professors could have their own overviews of what was going on in the field. "That's almost impossible today," she said, "with some 350 papers coming out daily now related to nutrition issues." Conducting systematic reviews were new to most of the approximately 100 nutrition experts who were involved in this last edition. Thus, it was a huge undertaking. In the process, they realized how challenging it was, with many pitfalls. "We probably went into every ditch that it is possible to go into on the road," she said. But they managed, in the end, to produce about 20 systematic reviews, which, after peer review, were published in the journal *Food and Nutrition Research*. The reviews were fed into the central working group and used as a basis for the recommendations. For Meltzer, this was a "sunshine story" of five countries who have been working together for many years.

Additionally, the two most recent Nordic nutrition recommendation revisions (i.e., the 2004 and 2012 editions) have included not only "go-throughs" of nutrients, but also dietary guidelines. Both also have included physical activity recommendations. Plus, the last edition contains chapters on what Meltzer called "hot topics" that do not necessarily apply to specific nutrients, but are pressing public issues (e.g., diet and sustainability).

Regarding challenges to global harmonization, Meltzer commented on the many pitfalls, the knowledge of biases required, and what she described as the humongous volumes of publications that need to be searched when conducting a systematic review. She suggested that systematic reviews be established as a specific specialty for students at the Ph.D. level. She described how most of the review committee members conducted the systematic review work on their own free time, and many worked unpaid. So the process was quite slow. "If this is to be feasible," she said, "I really think it should be a specialty in its own right. That's one of the learning points from our work."

In closing, she referred to the many challenges faced by EFSA, as described by Przyrembel. "Every one of those points would apply to the Nordic countries as well," she said.

SOUTHEAST ASIA[6]

In the past 4 years, several countries in Southeast Asia have revised their recommendations on nutrient intake. Emorn Udomkesmalee discussed these recommendations, emphasizing differences among countries, For example, in the case of recommended protein intake (grams/day), for the age group of 6–9 years, the levels range from 49 (Indonesia 2014) to 29–30

---

[6] This section summarizes information presented by Emorn Udomkesmalee, Ph.D., senior advisor, Mahidol University Institute of Nutrition, Thailand.

(Philippines 2015) to 32–33 (Vietnam 2016) to 12 (Malaysia 2017) (Personal communication, Professor Poh Bee Koon, Universiti Kebangsaan Malaysia). In Udomkesmalee's opinion, considering that these countries are in the same Association of Southeast Asian Nations (ASEAN) region, the average requirements for similar age ranges should not differ this much for any particular nutrient, including protein. She remarked that the wide variation seems to reflect different "judgments."

While the stepwise process to derive recommended nutrient intake is similar across countries, different countries follow different sets of existing international recommendations (e.g., the IOM, United Nations' Food and Agriculture Organization [FAO]/WHO, EFSA, the United Kingdom) depending on the preference of the country committee. Udomkesmalee explained that most of the national committees are assembled with expertise from broad and overarching areas in nutrition, food, and health-related disciplines and that very few members have expertise in in-depth, nutrient-specific areas of knowledge.

Another challenge is the limitation of quality data to help with decision making. Udomkesmalee speculated that a systematic review of locally available data to screen for the strength of evidence, based upon the previously mentioned criteria,[7] would reveal an urgent need to strengthen the quality of data. As an example, she cited controversy around the vitamin A bioconversion factor in the ongoing revision of Thailand Dietary Reference Intakes (DRIs). In 2003, the Thailand DRI committee adopted the IOM recommendation for a retinol activity equivalent bioconversion factor of 12:1 for beta-carotene (i.e., 12 μg of beta-carotene = 1 μg retinol [active form of vitamin A]), based on the evidence at that time from plant-based diets in developing countries. However, since then, as new data have become available, an EFSA panel has decided to maintain the older recommendation of a 6:1 bioconversion factor. According to Udomkesmalee, the Thailand DRI committee is not willing to adjust their current bioconversion factor because, as they see it, the new evidence is controversial and there is no international consensus yet regarding which factor suits what context. In addition, changing the bioconversion factor from 12:1 to 6:1 would require substantial efforts to correct all the raw data in the current national database.

A final challenge, Udomkesmalee continued, is that the DRIs are set for healthy populations, yet, for example, a significant proportion of the Thai population carries a thalassemia trait, which should be considered when setting the DRI for iron. In conclusion, Udomkesmalee emphasized the

---

[7] In session 2, "Exploring Approaches to Evaluating the Evidence," as summarized in Chapter 5.

critical need for guiding principles that the DRI committees can use when there is no clear "yes or no" decision.

DISCUSSION

Following their presentations, the panelists participated in an open discussion with the workshop audience, as summarized here.

Africa: Lack of Resources

Anura Kurpad asked "what went wrong" with the effort initiated to harmonize efforts in Africa and, if a similar effort is to be resumed, which institution or institutions would be plausible leaders. Ntambi responded that there are a number of organizations in African countries whose core function is nutrition, such as the National Food and Nutritional Council in Uganda. These organizations began collecting data some time back, he said, but a lack of resources led them to "getting stuck." If resources were to become available, that effort could be revived.

Additionally, Ntambi emphasized that most countries in Africa have national academies of sciences, and the academies have a lot of expertise in computer science, mathematics, and nutrition. If these experts were given the charge or task to conduct these evaluations, they should be able to do it, in his opinion. He suggested encouraging the African academies to hold workshops like this one, but on the African continent, and to begin discussing harmonization. "The expertise could be there," he said, "but the resources are lacking."

While on the topic of resources, Matthys added that many resources are donor driven, not necessarily needs driven, and that this needs to be taken into account. Additionally, he mentioned the issue of research waste and the need to reduce the "double-work" that many people do.

Nutrient Recommendation Values in the Nordic Countries

It appears that there is agreement around the vitamin D NRV among the Nordic countries, Peter Clifton observed, but disagreement around how to apply these values in practice, that is, whether via fortification or supplementation. He asked, has there been any discussion around the public health application of the vitamin D NRV in the different Nordic countries? Meltzer responded that the decision on how to implement recommended NRVs is left to the separate countries. Regarding the actual recommendations, she noted that there are only 2–3 nutrients with slight differences among countries. Most are exactly the same.

The Nordic Countries: Barriers and Lessons Learned

When asked by Laura Martino what barriers the Nordic countries have come up against and lessons learned, Meltzer mentioned the same list that Przyrembel had described for EFSA. She commented that, early on, they agreed that they should use systematic literature reviews. But because none of them were experienced with those, they enlisted the help of professional librarians. One of the biggest challenges within the review itself, she said, was that they started with two large questions that covered "everything" and had to narrow the questions quite substantially to make them "doable." She described the new literature that is emerging all the time as overwhelming, at least it was for the issues they decided to address, like vitamin D and fatty acids. Quality assessment was another challenge, she added, that is, "being able to really grasp the aspects of quality." They ended up using an A, B, C, or D quality grading system, one used by the World Cancer Research Fund International. Hardly any study received full marks, she noted.

Meltzer emphasized again, as she had during her talk, the need to have experienced people conducting systematic reviews. "It should become a specialty in its own right within the nutrition society," she urged, the kind of specialty that Ph.D. students or postdoctoral students work on, given its demanding nature. Yet, she said, "All of us should know a bit about how to do it, to appreciate the work behind it."

Systematic Reviews

Most of the discussion during this session revolved around systematic reviews, beginning with Lindsay Allen asking, "How many systematic reviews do we need?" She questioned how many systematic reviews are really needed within each country. In her opinion, different systematic reviews do not yield very different numbers, perhaps with the exception of a few nutrients with criteria that one could "quibble about." She expressed concern that the systematic review process cannot be applied everywhere and that the expenditure of resources by some groups is perhaps not necessary. For example, is it necessary in Thailand, or could that committee use results from EFSA's work, for instance?

Matthys responded that one of the challenges is that the defined health outcome could be different from country to country. That is, a health outcome of relevance in one country may not be relevant in another. This is especially true with chronic disease outcomes, he added. Chizuru Nishida agreed with Matthys that systematic reviews address multiple health outcomes and that the reviews change based on the scope of the work and the endpoints being addressed. Depending on a country's priorities, one could focus on those reviews that include specific evidence of relevance.

Susan Fairweather-Tait pointed out that an interesting scientific experiment is under way with the National Academies conducting a review of sodium in parallel with EFSA conducting a separate review. As far as she was aware, they were examining virtually the same endpoints. But the National Academies may be using the Grading of Recommendations Assessment, Development and Evaluation (GRADE) system, while EFSA would be using a risk-of-bias tool. She expressed curiosity about how these two reviews will turn out and whether the results will conflict. She added that the Australian review of sodium was also available for comparison. "We don't want endless systematic reviews," she said. "We want updates, of course, but it shouldn't be a business. It should be a means to an end."

Regarding the systematic reviews themselves, Nishida emphasized the importance of transparency regarding how the quality of evidence is evaluated. She noted that, in the past, FAO and WHO used the same World Cancer Research Fund International grading system used by the Nordic countries, adapting it for both the 2002 update of dietary goals and the 2008 update of fats and fatty acids. Since 2010, however, WHO no longer uses that system. Instead, it uses the GRADE system, with the quality of evidence being ranked as high, moderate, low, or very low. Her understanding was that EFSA uses yet another classification system. Use of these different systems can cause problems. As an example, she mentioned Codex's coining of the term *generally accepted*, which she found very confusing. To her and her colleagues, "generally accepted" evidence did not seem like convincing evidence. She encouraged harmonizing the use of different terms to express the quality of evidence.

Following Nishida's comments, however, Przyrembel pointed out that, in EFSA, the *generally accepted* terminology is old language used by experts in a group who, according to their conscience and knowledge, reached a conclusion that was generally acceptable. EFSA's current assessment process involving systematic reviews does not use that language, Przyrembel said. Additionally, in its assessments, in addition to conducting its own systematic reviews, EFSA also makes use of existing systematic reviews.

Regarding the dissemination of existing systematic reviews, Nishida mentioned that, in fact, there is a database, the WHO e-Library of Evidence in Nutrition. In the guidelines section, she said, not only are the full systematic reviews that guided the guidelines available, but so too are related existing systematic reviews from Cochrane and other sources. She explained that WHO has started collaborating with Cochrane to provide not just a link to their reviews, but also summaries of existing Cochrane reviews so people who are interested, but do not have the time to read a 400-page Cochrane review, can still access that information.

With respect to relying on systematic reviews, in Clifton's opinion, the problem is with chronic disease. He mentioned the controversy around saturated and polyunsaturated fats and how the six or seven available systematic reviews (of cohort and intervention studies) yield very different answers despite ostensibly doing exactly the same thing with the same kind of question. The "real bias," he said, is in the selection or omission of studies. While Cochrane reviews justify very fully why they omit certain studies, a major problem with many systematic reviews in the literature is that they do not. Thus, different systematic reviews may reveal different answers, depending on the omission or selection of studies. Yet, all of these reviews are published in peer-reviewed journals, some quite high ranking, according to Clifton. Although saturated and polyunsaturated fats are a good example, there are going to be many more micro- and macronutrients with the same problem, he predicted.

Matthys referred to a recent article in *JAMA* on the misuse of meta-analysis in nutrition (Barnard et al., 2017). He agreed that the problem is not just with saturated fatty acids but also red meats. Some reviews, depending on what they have omitted, recommend eating more red meat. "Quality assurance," he agreed with others, "is one of the key issues to tackle."

Laura Martino suggested further research on this topic, that is, how to combine different detailed assessments and come up with an overall judgment. She urged building on the GRADE approach in a way that adjusts for biases, accounting for both the direction and magnitude of biases.

One of the challenges that Thailand and other countries are going to face, Udomkesmalee observed, is the need for a review of systematic reviews. With different reference agencies having different ways of grading quality of evidence, she asked, on what basis are you asking countries to choose? She described the 2003 dietary guidelines in Thailand as a "cocktail mix" of FAO, WHO, and IOM recommendations and predicted that the 2017 guidelines would be even more mixed. They will be the result of what she described as a "judgment decision" on the part of the eight working groups in Thailand, each group coming up with its own "favorite." She encouraged harmonization of all the "background noise" created by the multiple approaches being used to develop reference values and suggested that the reference agencies themselves talk around the usefulness and application of their work.

The Value of Stored Raw Data

Matthys remarked that, despite repeatedly insisting that EURRECA's data would be open access, in fact, if he were to look into one of his external hard drives, he suspected he would find a lot of stuff. He suggested that perhaps EFSA too has data on its shelves that sit, with nobody able to access them. In other words, he said, EURRECA's data are not just a collation of papers, but they also include stored raw data. Making raw data from different institutions publicly available would be very beneficial, in his opinion. Committees from different countries could examine those raw data first and determine whether they are relevant. It may simplify things, he suggested.

Moving Forward: The Idea of a Global Consultative Group

"I feel like we've opened Pandora's box," Janet King said. She expressed being depressed after hearing about the many barriers to harmonization and did not want to leave the meeting without thoughts about how to come back together and go forward. She wondered whether there was a way to set up a global consultative group on nutrient recommendations to serve as a resource for all countries and regions. Such a resource would allow countries to build on the experiences of others and to modify others' approaches, as necessary, to accommodate population differences and also to provide feedback so others can benefit.

Rather than feeling depressed, Joseph Lau said that he was heartened by this discussion. He shared with the workshop that this same issue around systematic reviews was addressed in the context of health care and medicine 20 years ago. It is new only to nutrition, he observed. He mentioned a 2017 *JAMA* commentary (Barnard et al., 2017) addressing the same problem that he himself addressed in a *Lancet* commentary 20 years ago. The message, he said, was the same: one answer does not tell the whole story. In his opinion, the challenge for nutrition is that the quality and information available from the primary studies are lacking. He interpreted this discussion as a call for better, more comprehensive reporting of information in the primary studies. "People are beginning to recognize the challenges and problems," he said, "which is the first step in addressing an issue."

Matthys expressed optimism as well. There are positive steps being taken, he said, such as the African Evidence Network, which aims to increase the use of evidence-based decision making in nutrition and health and involves trainings at many universities. Another example is the Joint Programming Initiative in Europe to make primary data available. While there is still a lot of work to do, he said, "I would like to look at the bright side."

9

Moving the Conversation Forward

This final chapter presents workshop planning committee chair Stephanie Atkinson's closing summary and her three strategic messages to send to the consensus committee.[1]

CHAIR'S CLOSING SUMMARY

In her closing summary, Stephanie Atkinson summarized what she described as a "very generous sharing of experiences," both good as well as challenging ones. She observed a great enthusiasm and collaborative spirit for harmonizing and was struck by the honesty with which different people talked about their own experiences. In her opinion, the next steps will be "to make things happen." Very briefly, she highlighted what she heard in each of the sessions that pertain to this.

In the first session on harmonization frameworks, summarized in Chapters 3 and 4, several participants provided some excellent examples of what has worked, but with challenges remaining. These challenges include the need for transparency, lack of standardization among endpoints, the difficulties of setting requirements based on chronic disease, the need for a central repository for evidence, and variation in terminology. She remarked

[1] As previously mentioned, this workshop will help to inform a separate consensus effort to review and assess methodological approaches to developing nutrient intake recommendations: http://nationalacademies.org/hmd/Activities/Nutrition/NutrientIntakeRecommendations.aspx (accessed April 25, 2018).

that these same issues were mentioned or discussed throughout the workshop and will need to be addressed up front.

In session 2, on approaches to evaluating the evidence and summarized in Chapter 5, Atkinson perceived great hope that the field is on the brink of new, nutrition-specific methodology such that nutrition scientists will not have to think about how to apply their work to pharmaceutical trials. She especially liked Joseph Lau's quote, "Evidence is global, decision is local." In these days of open access and big data, she said, "Sharing is what it's about."

As summarized in Chapter 6, the discussion became more country specific in session 3, she observed, when contextual factors were addressed, although probably not for genetics or physiology. "We just need to recognize where [genetics and physiology] may be important factors," she said. For example, with respect to physiology, she referred to Anura Kurpad's discussion of the importance of understanding and accounting for adaptation when conducting randomized clinical trials. Atkinson referred to what she described as the two wonderful examples of health status indicators that vary among countries or regions: aging and infection. Aging is a global issue, affecting every country. Infection is more of a regional issue, she observed. Nonetheless, she suggested that perhaps there can be a global approach to recognizing the effects of infection on setting nutrient recommendations. Like infection, bioavailability has very different effects depending on the region. In her opinion, Rosalind Gibson and Umi Fahmida provided hope that new and more universal approaches are becoming available for assessing bioavailability.

Regarding the session 4 breakout discussions summarized in Chapter 7, Atkinson referred workshop participants to Lindsay Allen's summary at the end of that session. "We heard time and time again that the greatest advantage we can have is a central repository of evidence," she said. Yet, she added, there are still some needs that are more of an issue in some countries than in others, such as the need for good composition tables and dietary assessments at the population level. One of the greatest challenges is the disparate availability of resources among countries, she remarked. By sharing resources, such disparities could be alleviated.

Finally, in session 5 and summarized in Chapter 8, when representatives from different parts of the world shared their different experiences, the lack of a consistent approach to assessing the literature emerged as a major issue, with different systematic reviews following different protocols and different committees using different tools. Consistency will require standardizing these critical elements of the process, Atkinson said.

CHAIR'S THREE STRATEGIC MESSAGES

Atkinson identified three strategic messages to send to the consensus committee:

1. Develop a standardized methodological approach: "We would value a standardized methodological approach with rigorous scientific review of the literature," Atkinson said. Preferably, she added, this would be a centralized collaborative open for all countries to access. She referred to King's concept of a global consultative group on nutrient recommendations, as summarized at the end of Chapter 8, and suggested that perhaps the United Nations' Food and Agriculture Organization (FAO) or the World Health Organization (WHO) consider organizing such a group. She added that nutrition-specific tools, such as for risk of bias, and acceptance of standardized terminology would also be of great advantage. Regarding terminology, she acknowledged that different countries may not want to stop using their own terms, as reeducating the public would be difficult. She suggested, however, that at least the definitions be standardized such that regardless of what a value is called, all of its names have the same meaning.
2. Recognize the special needs of geographic regions or countries: Atkinson called for recognition of the special needs of geographic regions, or countries, related to food composition, dietary surveys, bioavailability, and health status.
3. Fill knowledge gaps: There is a desperate need to fill knowledge gaps and improve the science upon which to derive nutritional requirements that include phenotypic differences across the world, Atkinson stated. In her opinion, this is an area where the nutrition field needs to approach funding agencies. She expressed uncertainty around how to make an impact on funders, at least at the federal levels (e.g., National Institutes of Health, Canadian Institutes of Health Research), but said, "Let's not stop trying."

Finally, Atkinson suggested, as a first next step, a scoping of already completed work, such as the methodological work in process at WHO and available work on systematic reviews and other protocols, perhaps through the aforementioned global consultative group. She wondered if all of the knowledge accrued thus far could be combined under one tent, from which next steps could then be decided. "I do feel this isn't the end," she said. "It's only the beginning."

The workshop's parting words were provided by Francesco Branca, director of the WHO Department of Nutrition for Health and Development, who expressed gratitude to the National Academies for highlighting the challenge and persuading WHO and FAO to take it on. It is a "big gap area," he said, and it is not acceptable that such an important element, nutrient intake recommendations, which has both research and public health implications, has so many divergences not grounded in real biological or dietary differences, rather differences in interpretation, methodology, and terminology. His hope was that the understanding, or scoping, of the issues made possible by this workshop would help to move this field forward, although he also expressed caution given the complexity and magnitude of the challenge. We are "humbly here," he said, and will build on "what you have started to construct today."

References

Abrams, S. A. 2010. Setting Dietary Reference Intakes with the use of bioavailability data: Calcium. *American Journal of Clinical Nutrition* 91(5):1474S–1477S.*

AHRQ (Agency for Healthcare Research and Quality). 2008–2017 (living document). *Methods guide for effectiveness and comparative effectiveness reviews.* https://www.ncbi.nlm.nih.gov/books/NBK47095 (accessed December 21, 2017).

Alvarez, J. O., E. Salazar-Lindo, J. Kohatsu, P. Miranda, and C. B. Stephensen. 1995. Urinary excretion of retinol in children with acute diarrhea. *American Journal of Clinical Nutrition* 61(6):1273–1276.

Aung-Than-Batu, Thein-Than, and Thane-Toe. 1976. Iron absorption from Southeast Asian rice-based meals. *American Journal of Clinical Nutrition* 29:219–225.

Australian Government Department of Health. 2015. *Methodological framework for the review of nutrient reference values.* https://www.nrv.gov.au/sites/default/files/content/resources/Methodological%20Framework%2007032017%20CC4_0%20%284%29.pdf (accessed November 20, 2017).

Bai, A., V. K. Shukla, G. Bak, and G. Wells. 2012. *Quality assessment tools project report.* Ottawa, Canada: Canadian Agency for Drugs and Technologies in Health.

Barnard, N. E., W. C. Willett, and E. L. Ding. 2017. The misuse of meta-analysis in nutrition research. *JAMA*. doi:10.1001/jama.2017.12083.

Beisel, W. R., Y. F. Herman, H. E. Sauberlich, R. H. Herman, P. J. Bartelloni, and J. E. Canham. 1972. Experimentally induced sandfly fever and vitamin metabolism in man. *American Journal of Clinical Nutrition* 25(11):1165–1173.

Bostian, K. A., B. S. Blackburn, R. W. Wannemacher, Jr., V. G. McGann, W. R. Beisel, and H. L. Dupont. 1976. Sequential changes in the concentration of specific serum proteins during typhoid fever infection in man. *Journal of Laboratory and Clinical Medicine* 87(4):577–585.

---

* References with an asterisk (*) were not actually cited during the workshop and are therefore not cited anywhere in the text of this proceedings, but were included in the background bibliography distributed prior to the workshop.

Bow, C. H., E. Cheung, C. L. Cheung, S. M. Xiao, C. Loong, C. Soong, K. C. Tan, M. M. Luckey, J. A. Cauley, S. Fujiwara, and A. W. Kung. 2012. Ethnic difference of clinical vertebral fracture risk. *Osteoporosis International* 23(3):879–885.

Bresnahan, K. A., and S. A. Tanumihardjo. 2014. Undernutrition, the acute phase response to infection, and its effects on micronutrient status indicators. *Advances in Nutrition* 5(6):702–711.

Bresnahan, K. A., J. Chileshe, and S. A. Tanumihardjo. 2014. Quantification of food and nutrient intakes in Zambian children with and without malaria under controlled feeding conditions. *Experimental Biology and Medicine* 239(1):45–51.

Brown, K. A., M. Hermoso, L. Timotijevic, J. Barnett, I. T. Lillegaard, I. Řehůřková, A. Larrañaga, A. Lončarević-Srmić, L. F. Andersen, J. Ruprich, L. Fernández-Celemín, and M. M. Raats. 2013. Consumer involvement in dietary guideline development: Opinions from European stakeholders. *Public Health Nutrition* 16(5):769–776.

Brown, K. H., R. Y. Stallings, H. C. de Kanashiro, G. Lopez de Romaña, and R. E. Black, 1990. Effects of common illnesses on infants' energy intakes from breast milk and other foods during longitudinal community-based studies in Huascar (Lima), Peru. *American Journal of Clinical Nutrition* 52(6):1005–1013.

Campbell, W. W., M. C. Crim, G. E. Dallal, V. R. Young, and W. J. Evans. 1994. Increased protein requirements in elderly people: New data and retrospective assessments. *American Journal of Clinical Nutrition* 60(4):501–509.

Campbell, W. W., T. A. Trappe, R. R. Wolfe, and W. J. Evans. 2001. The recommended dietary allowance for protein may not be adequate for older people to maintain skeletal muscle. *Journal of Gerontology, Series A, Biological Science and Medical Sciences* 56(6):M373–M380.

Campos, F. A., H. Flores, and B. A. Underwood. 1987. Effect of an infection on vitamin A status of children as measured by the relative dose response (RDR). *American Journal of Clinical Nutrition* 46(1):91–94.

Castaneda, C., J. M. Charnley, W. J. Evans, and M. C. Crim. 1995. Elderly women accommodate to a low-protein diet with losses of body cell mass, muscle function, and immune response. *American Journal of Clinical Nutrition* 62(1):30–39.

Cavelaars, A. E., E. L. Doets, R. A. Dhonukshe-Rutten, M. Hermoso, S. J. Fairweather-Tait, B. Koletzko, M. Gurinović, L. A. Moreno, I. Cetin, C. Matthys, P. van 't Veer, M. Ashwell, and C. P. de Groot. 2010. Prioritizing micronutrients for the purpose of reviewing their requirements: A protocol developed by EURRECA. *European Journal of Clinical Nutrition* 64(Suppl 2):S19–S30.

CDC (Centers for Disease Control and Prevention). 2013. *The state of aging and health in America 2013*. Atlanta, GA: CDC. https://www.cdc.gov/aging/pdf/State-Aging-Health-in-America-2013.pdf (accessed November 20, 2017).

Chung, M., E. M. Balk, S. Ip, G. Raman, W. W. Yu, T. A. Trikalinos, A. H. Lichtenstein, E. A. Yetley, and J. Lau. 2009a. Reporting of systematic reviews of micronutrients and health: A critical appraisal. *American Journal of Clinical Nutrition* 89:1099–1113.

Chung, M., E. M., Balk, M. Brendel, S. Ip, J. Lau, J. Lee, A. Lichtenstein, K. Patel, G. Raman, A. Tatsioni, T. Terasawa, T. A. Trikalinos. 2009b. *Vitamin D and calcium: Systematic review of health outcomes*. Evidence Report/Technology Assessment No. 183. (AHRQ Publication No. 09-E015). Rockville, MD: Agency for Healthcare Research and Quality. https://www.ahrq.gov/downloads/pub/evidence/pdf/vitadcal/vitadcal.pdf (accessed February 9, 2018).

Crider, K. S., O. Devine, L. Hao, N. F. Dowling, S. Li, A. M. Molloy, Z. Li, J. Zhu, and R. J. Berry. 2014. Population red blood cell folate concentrations for prevention of neural tube defects: Bayesian model. *BMJ* 349:g4554.

Daly, L. E., P. N. Kirke, A. Molloy, D. G. Weir, and J. M. Scott. 1995. Folate levels and neural tube defects. Implications for prevention. *JAMA* 274(21):1698–1702.

Dhanwal, D. K., E. M. Dennison, N. C. Harvey, and C. Cooper. 2011. Epidemiology of hip fracture: Worldwide geographic variation. *Indian Journal of Orthopaedics* 45(1):15–22.

Dhonukshe-Rutten, R. A., J. Bouwman, K. A. Brown, A. E. Cavelaars, R. Collings, E. Grammatikaki, L. C. de Groot, M. Gurinović, L. J. Harvey, M. Hermoso, R. Hurst, B. Kremer, J. Ngo, R. Novakovi, M. M. Raats, F. Rolling, L. Serra-Majem, O. W. Souverein, L. Timotijevic, and P. van 't Veer. 2013. EURRECA-evidence-based methodology for deriving micronutrient recommendations. *Critical Reviews in Food Science and Nutrition* 53(10):999–1040.

Dosseter, J. F., and H. C. Whittle 1975. Protein-losing enteropathy and malabsorption in acute measles enteritis. *BMJ* 2(5971):592–593.

Duggan, M. B. and R. D. Milner. 1986. The maintenance energy requirement for children: An estimate based on a study of children with infection associated underfeeding. *American Journal of Clinical Nutrition* 43(6):870–878.

EFSA (European Food Safety Authority). 2015. Principles and process for dealing with data and evidence. *EFSA Journal* 13(5):4121. http://www.efsa.europa.eu/en/efsajournal/pub/4121 (accessed November 21, 2017).

EFSA. 2017a. *Dietary reference values for nutrients. Summary report.* EFSA Supporting Publication 2017:e15121. http://onlinelibrary.wiley.com/doi/10.2903/sp.efsa.2017.e15121/epdf (accessed February 16, 2018).

EFSA. 2017b. Guidance on the use of the weight of evidence approach in scientific assessments. *EFSA Journal* 15(8):4971.

EFSA NDA (European Food Safety Authority Panel on Dietetic Products, Nutrition, and Allergies). 2010. Principles for deriving and applying dietary reference values. *EFSA Journal* 8(3):1458. http://www.efsa.europa.eu/en/efsajournal/pub/1458 (accessed January 19, 2018).

EFSA NDA. 2014. Scientific opinion on dietary reference values for zinc. *EFSA Journal* 12(1):3844.

Ensrud, K. E. 2013. Epidemiology of fracture risk with advancing age. *Journal of Gerontology, Series A, Biological Sciences and Medical Sciences* 68(10):1236–1242.

Fairweather-Tait, S. J., and R. Collings. 2010. Estimating the bioavailability factors needed for setting dietary reference values. *International Journal for Vitamin and Nutrition Research* 80(4):249–256.*

Fan, S., M. E. Hansen, Y. Lo, and S. A. Tishkoff. 2016. Going global by adapting loci: A review of recent human evolution. *Science* 354(6308):54–59.

FAO (Food and Agriculture Organization). 2013. *Dietary protein quality evaluation in human nutrition.* Food and Nutrition Paper 92. http://www.fao.org/ag/humannutrition/35978-02317b979a686a57aa4593304ffc17f06.pdf (accessed February 16, 2018).

FAO/WHO (World Health Organization). 1998. *Preparation and use of food-based dietary guidelines.* http://www.fao.org/docrep/X0243E/x0243e00.htm (accessed November 20, 2017).

FAO/WHO. 2017. *Global Individual Food consumption data Tool (GIFT): Project brief.* http://www.fao.org/fileadmin/user_upload/nutrition/docs/assessment/2017-08-10_FAO-WHO_GIFT_Briefing_document_mod.pdf (accessed December 21, 2017).

Fiatarone, M. A., E. F. O'Neill, N. D. Ryan, K. M. Clements, G. R. Solares, M. E. Nelson, S. B. Roberts, J. J. Kehayias, L. A. Lipsitz, and W. J. Evans. 1994. Exercise training and nutritional supplementation for physical frailty in very elderly people. *New England Journal of Medicine* 330(25):1769–1775.

Flores-Ayala, R., and S. Fairweather-Tait. 2012. *Human zinc requirements: Report of the HarvestPlus consultation on physiological and dietary zinc requirements*. http://nationalacademies.org/hmd/~/media/Files/Activity%20Files/Global/2017-sept-21-GlobalHarmonizationofMethod/3%20Harvest%20Plus%20Zinc%20Consultation.pdf?la=en (accessed December 21, 2017).*

Forsythe, L. K., M. B. Livingstone, M. S. Barnes, G. Horigan, E. M. McSorley, M. P. Bonham, P. J. Magee, T. R. Hill, A. J. Lucey, K. D. Cashman, M. Kiely, J. J. Strain, and J. M. Wallace. 2012. Effect of adiposity on vitamin D status and the 25-hydroxycholecalciferol response to supplementation in healthy young and older Irish adults. *British Journal of Nutrition* 107(1):126–134.

Fredriksen, A., K. Meyer, P. M. Ueland, S. E. Voliset, T. Grotmol, and J. Schneede. 2007. Large-scale population-based metabolic phenotyping of thirteen genetic polymorphisms related to one-carbon metabolism. *Human Mutation* 28(9):856–865.

Ghadimi H., S. Kumar, and F. Abaci. 1973. Endogenous amino acid loss and its significance in infantile diarrhea. *Pediatric Research* 7(3):161–168.

Gibson, R. S. 2007. The role of diet- and host-related factors in nutrient bioavailability and thus in nutrient-based dietary requirement estimates. *Food and Nutrition Bulletin* 28(1):S77–S100.*

Gibson, R. S. 2012. Harmonisation of micronutrient-based dietary standards globally: Challenges and future developments. *Nutrition & Dietetics* 69(3):183–186.*

Haddad, J. G., L. Y. Matsuoka, B. W. Hollis, Y. Z. Hu, and J. Wortsman. 1993. Human plasma transport of vitamin D after its endogenous synthesis. *Journal of Clinical Investigation* 91(6):2552–2555.

Hallberg, L., L. Garby, R. Suwanik, and E. Björn-Rasmussen. 1974. Iron absorption from Southeast Asian diets. *American Journal of Clinical Nutrition* 27(8):826–836.

Hallberg, L., E. Björn-Rasmussen, L. Rossander, and R. Suwanik. 1977. Iron absorption from Southeast Asian diets. II. Role of various factors that might explain low absorption. *American Journal of Clinical Nutrition* 30(4):539–548.

Higgins, J. P. T., and S. Green (eds.). 2011. *Cochrane handbook for systematic reviews of interventions*. Version 5.1.0. http://training.cochrane.org/handbook (accessed December 21, 2017).

Hoekstra, J., J. Verkaik-Kloosterman, C. Rompelberg, H. van Kranen, M. Zeilmaker, H. Verhagen, and N. de Jong. 2007. Integrated risk-benefit analyses: Method development with folic acid as example. *Food and Chemical Toxicology* 46:893–909.

Holick, M. F. 2012. The D-lightful vitamin D for child health. *Journal of Parenteral and Enteral Nutrition* 36(1 Suppl):9S–19S.

Houston, D. K., B. J. Nicklas, J. Ding, T. B. Harris, F. A. Tylavsky, A. B. Newman, J. S. Lee, N. R. Sahyoun, M. Visser, and S. B. Kritchevsky, and Health ABC Study. 2008. Dietary protein intake is associated with lean mass change in older, community-dwelling adults; the Health, Aging, and Body Composition (Health ABC) Study. *American Journal of Clinical Nutrition* 87(1):150–155.

Hunt, J. R., and Z. K. Roughead. 2000. Adaptation of iron absorption in men consuming diets with high or low iron bioavailability. *American Journal of Clinical Nutrition* 71(1):94–102.*

Hurrell, R. F., S. Lynch, T. Bothwell, H. Cori, R. Glahn, E. Hertrampf, Z. Kratky, D. Miller, M. Rodenstein, H. Streekstra, B. Teucher, E. Turner, C. K. Yeung, M. B. Zimmermann, and Sharing United States Technology to Aid in the Improvement of Nutrition (SUSTAIN) Task Force. 2004. Enhancing the absorption of fortification iron—A SUSTAIN Task Force report. *International Journal for Vitamin and Nutrition Research* 74(6):387–401.

ILSI (International Life Sciences Institute, Southeast Asia Region). 2005. *Recommended dietary allowances: Harmonization in Southeast Asia.* http://ilsisea-region.org/wp-content/uploads/sites/21/2016/06/ILSI-SEAR-Monograph-ASEAN-RDAs.pdf (accessed February 16, 2018).

IOM (Institute of Medicine). 1994. *How should the recommended dietary allowances be revised?* Washington, DC: National Academy Press.

IOM. 2002. *Dietary Reference Intakes: Energy, carbohydrates, fiber, fat, fatty acids, cholesterol, protein, and amino acids.* Washington, DC: The National Academies Press.

IOM. 2005. *Dietary Reference Intakes for water, potassium, sodium, chloride, and sulfate.* Washington, DC: The National Academies Press.

IOM. 2011a. *Dietary Reference Intakes for calcium and vitamin D.* Washington, DC: The National Academies Press.

IOM. 2011b. *Finding what works in health care: Standards for systematic reviews.* Washington, DC: The National Academies Press.

Itan, Y., B. L. Jones, C. J. E. Ingram, D. M. Swallow, and M. G. Thomas. 2010. A worldwide correlation of lactase persistence phenotype and genotypes. *BMC Evolutionary Biology* 10:36.

Janssen, I., S. B. Heymsfield, Z. M. Wang, and R. Ross. 2000. Skeletal muscle mass and distribution in 468 men and women aged 18–88 yr. *Journal of Applied Physiology* 89(1):81–88.

Jeruszka-Bielak, M., E. Sicińska, L. de Wit, J. Ruprich, I. Řehůřková, K. A. Brown, L. Timotijevic, A.-M. Sonne, P. Haugaard, A. Guzzon, N. B. Garcia, E. Alevritou, M. Hermoso, Y. Sarmant, L. Lähteenmäki, W. Roszkowski, and M. M. Raats. 2015. Stakeholders' views on factors influencing nutrition policy: A qualitative study across ten European countries. *Polish Journal of Food and Nutrition Sciences* 65(4):293–302.*

Kenney, A. M., and K. M. Prestwood. 2000. Osteoporosis: Pathogenesis, diagnosis, and treatment in older adults. *Rheumatic Disease Clinics of North America* 26(3):569–591.

King, J. C., and C. Garza (Eds). 2007. International harmonization of approaches for developing nutrient-based dietary standards. *Food and Nutrition Bulletin* 28(1):S1–S153.

Kocher, A. R. 1914. Über die größe des eiweißzerfalls bei fieber und bei arbeitsleistung. *Deutsches Archiv Fur Klinische Medizin* 115:82 [article in German].

Kumssa, D. B., E. J. Joy, E. L. Ander, M. J. Watts, S. D. Young, S. Walker, and M. R. Broadley. 2015. Dietary calcium and zinc deficiency risks are decreasing but remain prevalent. *Scientific Reports* 5:10974.

Kwun, I. S., and C. S. Kwon. 2000. Dietary molar ratios of phytate:zinc and millimolar ratios of phytate x calcium:zinc in South Koreans. *Biological Trace Element Research* 75(1–3):29–41.

Leonard, W. R. 2002. Food for thought: Dietary change was a driving force in human evolution. *Scientific American* 287(6):106–115.

Lupton, J. R., S. A. Atkinson, N. Chan, C. G. Fraga, J. Levy, M. Messina, D. P. Richardson, B. van Ommen, Y. Yang, and J. C. Griffiths. 2014. Exploring the benefits and challenges of establishing a DRI-like process for bioactives. *European Journal of Nutrition* 53(1):1–9.*

Ma, G., Y. Li, Y. Jin, F. Zhai, F. J. Kok, and X. Yang. 2007. Phytate intake and molar ratios of phytate to zinc, iron and calcium in the diets of people in China. *European Journal of Clinical Nutrition* 61(3):368–374.

Ma, J., M. J. Stampfer, B. Christensen, E. Giovannucci, D. J. Hunter, J. Chen, W. C. Willett, J. Selhub, C. H. Hennekens, R. Gravel, and R. Rozen. 1999. A polymorphism of the methionine synthase gene: Association with plasma folate, vitamin B12, homocyst(e)ine, and colorectal cancer risk. *Cancer Epidemiology, Biomarkers & Prevention* 8(9):825–829.

MacCallum, W. G. 1910. Fever, in *The Harvey Lectures, Volume 4*. Philadelphia, PA: J.B. Lippincott Co.

Martorell, R., C. Yarbrough, S. Yarbrough, and R. E. Klein. 1980. The impact of ordinary illnesses on the dietary intakes of malnourished children. *American Journal of Clinical Nutrition* 33(2):345–350.

Matthys, C., L. Bucchini, M. C. Busstra, A. E. J. M. Cavelaars, P. Eleftherious, A. Garcia-Alvarez, S. Fairweather-Tait, M. Gurinovic, B. Van Ommen, and L. Contor. 2010. EURRECA: Development of tools to improve the alignment of micronutrient recommendations. *European Journal of Clinical Nutrition* 64(S3):S26–S31.*

Miller, L. V., N. F. Krebs, and K. M. Hambidge. 2007. A mathematical model of zinc absorption in humans as a function of dietary zinc and phytate. *Journal of Nutrition* 137:135–141.

Mithal, A., D. A. Wahl., J.-P. Bonjour, P. Burckhardt, B. Dawson-Huges, J. A. Eisman, G. El-Haajj Fuleihan, R. G. Josse, P. Lips, and J. Morales-Torres. 2009. Global vitamin D and determinants of hypovitaminosis D. *Osteoporosis International* 20(11):1807–1820.*

Mitra, A. K., J. O. Alvarez, L. Guay-Woodford, G. J. Fuchs, M. A. Wahed, and C. B. Stephensen. 1998. Urinary retinol excretion and kidney function in children with shigellosis. *American Journal of Clinical Nutrition* 68(5):1095–1103.

Molla, A., A. M. Molla, A. Rahim, S. A. Sarker, Z. Mozaffar, and M. Rahaman. 1982. Intake and absorption of nutrients in children with cholera and rotavirus infection during acute diarrhea and after recovery. *Nutrition Research* 2(3):233–242.

Narasinga Rao, B. S., C. Vijayasarathy, and T. Prabhavathi. 1983. Iron absorption from habitual diets of Indians studied by the extrinsic tag technique. *Indian Journal of Medical Research* 77:648–657.

NASEM (National Academies of Sciences, Engineering, and Medicine). 2017a. *Guiding principles for developing Dietary Reference Intakes based on chronic disease.* Washington, DC: The National Academies Press.

NASEM. 2017b. *Redesigning the process for establishing the* Dietary Guidelines for Americans. Washington, DC: The National Academies Press.

National Center for Health Statistics. 2016. *Health, United States, 2015: With special features on racial and ethnic health disparities.* https://www.cdc.gov/nchs/hus/index.htm (accessed November 20, 2017).

Netherlands National Institute for Public Health and the Environment (RIVM). 2004. *Our Food, Our Health: Healthy Diet and Safe Food in the Netherlands.* http://www.rivm.nl/bibliotheek/rapporten/270555009.pdf (accessed December 12, 2017).

Nordic Council of Ministers. 2014. *Nordic nutrition recommendations 2012,* 5th ed. https://www.norden.org/en/theme/former-themes/themes-2016/nordic-nutrition-recommendation/nordic-nutrition-recommendations-2012 (accessed November 20, 2017).

Olhorst, S. D., R. Russell, D. Bier, D. M. Klurfeld, Z. Li, J. R. Mein, J. Milner, A. C. Ross, P. Sotver, and E. Konopka. 2013. Nutrition research to affect food and a healthy life span. *American Journal of Clinical Nutrition* 98(2):620–625.

Palacios, C., and L. Gonzalez. 2014. Is vitamin D deficiency a major global public health problem? *Journal of Steroid Biochemistry and Molecular Biology* 144(Pt A):138–145.

Pontzer, H., R. Durazo-Arvizu, L. R. Dugas, J. Plange-Rhule, P. Bovet, T. E. Forrester, E. V. Lambert, R. S. Cooper, D. A. Schoeller, and A. Luke. 2016. Constrained total energy expenditure and metabolic adaptation to physical activity in adult humans. *Current Biology* 26(3):410–417.

Quevedo, M. R., G. M. Price, D. Halliday, P. J. Pacy, and D. J. Millward. 1994. Nitrogen homeostasis in man: Diurnal changes in nitrogen excretion, leucine oxidation, and whole body leucine kinetics during a reduction from a high to a moderate protein intake. *Clinical Science* 86(2):185–193.

Reddy, V., N. Raghuramulu, Arunjyoti, M. Shivaprakash, and B. Underwood. 1986. Absorption of vitamin A by children with diarrhoea during treatment with oral rehydration salt solution. *Bulletin of the World Health Organization* 64(5):721–724.

Reeves, B. C., G. A. Wells, and H. Waddington. 2017. Quasi-experimental study designs series—paper 5: A checklist for classifying studies evaluating the effects of health interventions—a taxonomy without labels. *Journal of Clinical Epidemiology* 89:30–42.

Rosado, J. L., K. M. Hambidge, L. V. Miller, O. P. Garcia, J. Westcott, K. Gonzalez, J. Conde, C. Hotz, W. Pfeiffer, I. Ortiz-Monasterio, and N. F. Krebs. 2009. The quantity of zinc absorbed from wheat in adult women is enhanced by biofortification. *Journal of Nutrition* 139(10):1920–1925.

Russell, R., M. Chung, E. M. Balk, S. Atkinson, E. L. Giovannucci, S. Ip, A. H. Lichtenstein, S. T. Mayne, G. Raman, A. C. Ross, and T. A. Trikalinos. 2009. Opportunities and challenges in conducting systematic reviews to support the development of nutrient reference values: Vitamin A as an example. *American Journal of Clinical Nutrition* 89(3):728–733.

SCF (Scientific Committee for Food). 1993. Nutrient and energy intakes for the European Community. *Reports of the Scientific Committee for Food*, 31st Series. Luxembourg: Commission of the European Communities.

Scrimshaw, N. S. 1977. Effect of infection on nutrient requirements. *American Journal of Clinical Nutrition* 30(9):1536–1544.

Seeman, E. 2003. Invited review: Pathogenesis of osteoporosis. *Journal of Applied Physiology* 95(5):2142–2151.

Shea, B. J., J. M. Grimshaw, G. A. Wells, M. Boers, N. Andersson, C. Hamel, A. C. Porter, P. Tugwell, D. Moher, and L. M. Bouter. 2007. Development of AMSTAR: A measurement tool to assess the methodological quality of systematic reviews. *BMC Medical Research Methodology* 7:10.

Shea, B J., B C. Reeves, G. Wells, M. Thuku, C. Hamel, J. Moran, D. Moher, P. Tugwell, V. Welch, E. Kristjansson, and D. A. Henry. 2017. AMSTAR 2: A critical appraisal tool for systematic reviews that include randomised or non-randomised studies of healthcare interventions, or both. *British Medical Journal* 358:j4008.

Shetty, P. 2005. Energy requirements of adults. *Public Health Nutrition* 8(7a):994–1009.*

SIGN (Scottish Intercollegiate Guidelines Network). 2015. *SIGN 50: A guideline developer's handbook*. http://www.sign.ac.uk/checklists-and-notes.html (accessed February 1, 2018).

Solis, C., K. Veenema, A. A. Ivanov, S. Tran, R. Li, W. Wang, D. J. Moriarty, C. V. Maletz, and M. A. Caudill. 2008. Folate intake at RDA levels is inadequate for Mexican American men with the methylenetetrahydrofolate reductase 677TT genotype. *Journal of Nutrition* 138:67–72.

Stephensen, C. B., J. O. Alvarez, J. Kohatsu, R. Hardmeier, J. I. Kennedy, Jr., and R. B. Gammon, Jr. 1994. Vitamin A is excreted in the urine during acute infection. *American Journal of Clinical Nutrition* 60(3):388–392.

Sterne, J. A. C., M. A. Hernán, B. C. Reeves, J. Savović, and N. D. Berkman, M. Viswanathan, D. Henry, D. G. Altman, M. T. Ansari, I. Boutron, and J. R. Carpenter. 2016. ROBINS-1: A tool for assessing risk of bias in non-randomised studies of interventions. *British Medical Journal* 355:i4919.

Stover, P. J. 2007. Human nutrition and genetic variation. *Food and Nutrition Bulletin* 28(1 Suppl. International):S101–A115.

Threapleton, D. E., D. C. Greenwood, C. E. Evans, C. L. Cleghorn, C. Nykjaer, C. Woodhead, J. E. Cade, C. P. Gale, and V. J. Burlety. 2013. Dietary fibre intake and risk of cardiovascular disease: Systematic review and meta-analysis. *BMJ* 347:f6879.

Timotijevic, L., J. Barnett, and M. M. Raats. 2011. Engagement, representativeness and legitimacy in the development of food and nutrition policy. *Food Policy* 36(4):490–498.

Timotijevic, L., K. A. Brown, L. Lähteenmäki, L. de Wit, A. M. Sonne, J. Ruprich, I. Řehůřková, M. Jeruszka-Bielak, E. Sicinska, N. Brito Garcia, A. Guzzon, B. B. Jensen, R. Shepherd, J. Barnett, and M. M. Raats. 2013. EURRECA—A framework for considering evidence in public health nutrition policy development. *Critical Reviews in Food Science and Nutrition* 53(10):1124–1134.

U.S. Department of Energy. 2017. *Human Genome Project information archive, 1990–2003.* http://web.ornl.gov/sci/techresources/Human_Genome/index.shtml (accessed November 29, 2017).

van Buuren S., Y. Schönbeck, and P. van Dommelen. 2012. *Collection, collation and analysis of data in relation to reference heights and reference weights for female and male children and adolescents (0–18 years) in the EU, as well as in relation to the age of onset of puberty and the age at which different stages of puberty are reached in adolescents in the EU.* Final Report CT/EFSA/NDA/2010/01. EFSA Supporting Publications 2012:EN-255. http://onlinelibrary.wiley.com/doi/10.2903/sp.efsa.2012.EN-255/abstract (accessed January 19, 2018).

van Kreijl, C. F., and A. G. A. C. Knaap. 2004. *Ons eten gemeten: Gezonde voiding en veilig voedsel in Nederland.* No. 270555007. Bohn Stafleu van Loghum.

Wacker, M., and M. F. Holick. 2013. Sunlight and vitamin D: A global perspective for health. *Dermatoendocrinology* 5(1):51–108.

Wessells, K. R., and K. H. Brown. 2012. Estimating the global prevalence of zinc deficiency: Results based on zinc availability in national food supplies and the prevalence of stunting. *PLoS One* 7(11):e50568.

Wessells, K. R., G. M. Singh, and K. H. Brown. 2012. Estimating the global prevalence of inadequate zinc intake from national food balance sheets: Effects of methodological assumptions. *PLoS One* 7(11):e50565.

WHO (World Health Organization). 2010. *WHO global network of institutions for scientific advice on nutrition.* http://www.who.int/nutrition/publications/scientificadvice_global_network_institutions/en (accessed December 20, 2017).

WHO. 2015a. *Guideline. Optimal Serum and Red Blood Cell Folate Concentrations in Women of Reproductive Age for Prevention of Neural Tube Defects.* http://www.who.int/nutrition/publications/guidelines/optimalserum_rbc_womenrep_tubedefects/en (accessed November 21, 2017).

WHO. 2015b. *WHO estimates of the global burden of foodborne diseases.* http://www.who.int/foodsafety/publications/foodborne_disease/fergreport/en (accessed November 21, 2017).

WHO/FAO (Food and Agriculture Organization). 2004. *Vitamin and mineral requirements in human nutrition*, 2nd ed. http://apps.who.int/iris/bitstream/10665/42716/1/9241546123.pdf (accessed January 10, 2018).

WHO/FAO. 2005. *Model for establishing upper levels of intake for nutrients and related substances.* Report of a Joint FAO/WHO Technical Workshop on Nutrient Risk Assessment, WHO Headquarters, Geneva, Switzerland, 2-6 May, 2005. http://www.who.int/ipcs/methods/nra_final.pdf (accessed November 18, 2017).

Yetley, E. A., A. J. MacFarlane, L. S. Greene-Finestone, C. Garza, J. D. Ard, S. A. Atkinson, D. M. Bier, A. L. Carriquiry, W. R. Harlan, D. Hattis, J. C. King, D. Krewski, D. L. O'Connor, R. L. Prentice, J. V. Rodricks, and G. A. Wells. 2016. Options for basing Dietary Reference Intakes (DRIs) on chronic disease endpoints: Report from a joint US/Canadian-sponsored working group. *American Journal of Clinical Nutrition* 105(1):249S–285S.

Appendix A

Workshop Agenda

A WORKSHOP ON GLOBAL HARMONIZATION OF METHODOLOGICAL APPROACHES TO NUTRIENT INTAKE RECOMMENDATIONS

September 21–22, 2018
Headquarters of the Food and Agriculture Organization (FAO) of the United Nations
Viale delle Terme di Caracalla
Rome, Italy

WORKSHOP OBJECTIVES

- Describe potential frameworks to enable global harmonization of methodologies to establish nutrient intake recommendations.
- Explore approaches for evaluating the evidence to facilitate global harmonization of methodologies to establish nutrient intake recommendations.
- Examine the potential for addressing contextual factors from different population subgroups, regions, and countries that may or may not be conducive to harmonization.
- Consider approaches to facilitate global sharing of resources to maintain quality and support cost-effectiveness to develop methodologies for nutrient intake recommendations.
- Identify the advantages, barriers, and challenges to global harmonization of methodologies to establish nutrient intake recommendations.

DAY 1

8:30 am **Registration**

INTRODUCTION AND OPENING REMARKS

9:00 **Welcome**
Kostas Stamoulis, FAO Assistant Director-General, Economic and Social Development Department
Stephanie Atkinson, McMaster University, Planning Committee Chair

9:15 **Defining the Problem: Partner Panel**
- World Health Organization, *Chizuru Nishida, Coordinator, Nutrition Policy and Scientific Advice, Department of Nutrition for Health and Development*
- FAO, *Anna Lartey, Director of Nutrition*

9:30 **Background for the Workshop:**
Moderated by: Stephanie Atkinson, McMaster University, Planning Committee Chair

Harmonizing the Nutrient Intake Values: Phase 1
Janet King, Children's Hospital Oakland Research Institute

Applications and Uses of Nutrient Intake Recommendations
Suzanne Murphy, University of Hawaii

SESSION 1: HARMONIZATION FRAMEWORKS

Moderated by: Peter Clifton, University of South Australia

10:00 **Terminology and Models**
Peter Clifton, University of South Australia

10:20 **Endpoints—Deficiency Versus Chronic Disease**
Amanda MacFarlane, Health Canada

10:40 **Guiding Principles for Developing Dietary Reference Intakes Based on Chronic Disease**
Janet King, Children's Hospital Oakland Research Institute

10:50 **Discussion with Session Speakers**

11:10 **Break**

11:30 **Panel Discussion: Current Models for Establishing Intake Recommendations**
Canada: *Hasan Hutchinson, Health Canada, Panel Chair and Moderator*
United Kingdom: *Ann Prentice, University of Cambridge*
Australia and New Zealand: *Peter Clifton, University of South Australia*
South Korea: *Hee Young Paik, Seoul National University*

SESSION 2: APPROACHES TO EVALUATING THE EVIDENCE

Moderated by: Ann Prentice, University of Cambridge

12:10 pm **Tools for Evaluating Strength and Quality of Evidence**
George Wells, Ottawa Heart Institute

12:30 **Global Systematic Reviews: How Can It Be Done?**
Joseph Lau, Brown University

12:50 **Risk–Benefit Analysis**
Hans Verhagen, European Food Safety Authority (EFSA)

1:10 **Discussion with Session Speakers**

1:35 **Break for Lunch**

SESSION 3: CONTEXTUAL FACTORS: HOST, DIET/ ENVIRONMENT, AND HEALTH STATUS

Moderated by: Suzanne Murphy, Emerita, University of Hawaii, and John Muyonga, Makerere University

2:25 **The Role of Host: Genetic Variation**
Patrick Stover, Cornell University

2:45 **The Role of Host: Physiology**
Anura Kurpad, St. John's Medical College

3:05 **The Role of Health Status**
Seth Adu-Afarwuah, University of Ghana
Caryl Nowson, Deakin University

3:45 **The Role of Diet and Environment: Bioavailability, Processing, Environmental Exposure, and Nutrient Interactions**
Rosalind Gibson, University of Otago
Umi Fahmida, University of Indonesia

4:20 **Panel Discussion with Session Speakers**

4:50 **Closing Remarks**
Stephanie Atkinson, McMaster University, Planning Committee Chair

5:00 **Adjourn for the Day**

DAY 2

SESSION 4: APPLICATIONS, FACILITATING QUALITY, AND COST-EFFECTIVENESS

Moderated by: Lindsay Allen, University of California, Davis

8:30 am **Setting the Stage for Participant Discussion**
Catherine Leclercq, FAO

8:45 **Breakout Group Topics for Participant Discussion:**
- What are the advantages of global harmonization of methodologies for developing nutrient intake recommendations, from your standpoint?
- What additional resources and expertise would facilitate adoption of a harmonized approach in your region/country?
- What are the likely barriers and challenges to achieving global harmonization from your standpoint?

10:00 **Rapporteurs Report on Breakout Discussion**

10:30 **Break**

11:00 **Synthesis of Breakout Discussion**
Lindsay Allen, University of California, Davis

SESSION 5: ADVANTAGES, BARRIERS, AND CHALLENGES TO GLOBAL HARMONIZATION OF METHODOLOGIES FOR NUTRIENT INTAKE RECOMMENDATIONS

11:30 *Moderated by: Susan Fairweather-Tait, University of East Anglia, and Amanda MacFarlane, Health Canada*

Panel Discussion—Experiences from Countries That Have Collaborated

Countries/Entities Reporting:
Southeast Asia—Emorn Udomkesmalee, Mahidol University
European Micronutrient Recommendations Aligned (EURRECA)—Christophe Matthys, University of Leuven
EFSA—Hildegard Przyrembel, Federal Institute for Risk Assessment
Africa—James Ntambi, University of Wisconsin–Madison
Norway—Helle Margrete Meltzer, Norwegian Institute of Public Health

Topics for Discussion:
- Similarities and differences
- Challenges and advantages
- Mechanisms that could be considered for setting priorities for activities, such as systematic reviews, toolkits, technical briefs
- Potential for acceptance of methodological approaches across countries
- Potential ways forward

1:00 pm **Chair's Summary and Discussion of Next Steps**
Stephanie Atkinson, McMaster University, Planning Committee Chair

1:30 **Adjourn Meeting**

Appendix B

Speaker and Facilitator Biographies

Seth Adu-Afarwuah, Ph.D., is project manager at International Lipid Based Nutrient Supplements (iLiNS)-Ghana at the University of Ghana. Dr. Adu-Afarwuah's research is in the area of maternal and infant nutrition, with a focus on the prevention and treatment of malnutrition. His previous work includes the assessment of the efficacy and acceptability of multiple micronutrient supplements used in home fortification for pregnant and lactating women and infants, and the impact of lipid-based nutrient supplements given to children attending routine growth-monitoring sessions on prevention of severe acute malnutrition. Before the iLiNS Project, Dr. Adu-Afarwuah worked with the United Nations Children's Fund (UNICEF), first as a nutrition consultant and then as a nutrition program officer. He has also been a consultant for the World Bank. In the iLiNS Project, Dr. Adu-Afarwuah is the project manager for the Ghana site.

Lindsay Allen, Ph.D., has been the center director of the U.S. Department of Agriculture, Agricultural Research Service (USDA, ARS) Western Human Nutrition Research Center since 2004. She was formerly a professor in the Department of Nutrition at the University of California, Davis, where she is now an adjunct research professor. Dr. Allen's research focuses on the prevalence, causes, and consequences of micronutrient deficiencies, primarily in developing countries. She has evaluated interventions with micronutrient supplements, food fortification, and food-based approaches to improve nutritional status, pregnancy outcomes, and child development, resulting in more than 200 publications from many countries. One of her most important achievements has been to document the widespread high prevalence of vitamin B12 deficiency. Her research investigates the adverse functional consequences of this deficiency on infants, children, and women in developing countries, as well as the elderly in the United States, and the effects of different interventions to alleviate this deficiency. These interventions have included supplements for lactating women, infants, and children; animal source foods (meat and milk); and intramuscular injection of high doses. She is part of a team testing the use of 14C-vitamin B12, measured by accelerator mass spectrometry, for measuring vitamin B12 absorption and bioavailability in various conditions. Her laboratory is currently collaborating in the development and evaluation of a new combined indicator of vitamin B12 status, cB12. Dr. Allen's laboratory has recently developed efficient mass spectrometry and high-performance liquid chromatography methods for the measurement of multiple vitamins simultaneously in human milk. Application of these methods is revealing poor breast milk micronutrient content in some populations consuming poor quality diets, and enabling assessment of the effect of maternal supplementation on breast milk quality. Dr. Allen has served on 10 committees of the Food and Nutrition Board of the National Academies of Sciences, Engineering, and Medicine, including the Standing Committee on the Scientific Evaluation of Dietary Reference Intakes. She has advised many national, bilateral, and international organizations including World Health Organization (WHO), UNICEF, the Asian Development Bank, the World Bank, Pan American Health Organization (PAHO), and Food and Agriculture Organization (FAO). She is principal author of the book *What Works? A Review of the Efficacy and Effectiveness of Nutrition Interventions*, and of WHO's *Guidelines on Food Fortification with Micronutrients*. She served as president of the American Society of Nutritional Sciences and the Society for International Nutrition Research, and vice president of the International Union of Nutritional Sciences. From the American Society for Nutrition she received the Kellogg Prize for International Nutrition, the Conrad A. Elvehjem Award for Public Service in Nutrition, and the McCollum International Lectureship. Dr. Allen is currently a member of the steering committee of the Micronutrient Forum and the International Nutrition Foundation, and chair of the National Institutes of Health's (NIH's) Biomarkers in Nutrition and Development Expert Panel on Vitamin B12.

Stephanie Atkinson, Ph.D., D.Sc. (Hon), F.C.A.H.S., is tenured professor and nutrition clinician–scientist in the Department of Pediatrics, and associate member, Department of Biochemistry and Biomedical Sciences, Faculty of Health Sciences, McMaster University, as well as professional staff in McMaster Children's Hospital, Hamilton, Ontario, Canada. Her research has focused on pediatric nutrition, particularly in relation to skeletal development in premature and term infants and in children with boney morbidity secondary to disease process and/or drug therapy (e.g., steroids) in diseases such as lymphoblastic leukemia, nephrosis, rheumatoid disorders, cystic fibrosis, or epilepsy. Current research encompasses clinical trial and epidemiological investigations beginning in pregnancy that explore the environmental (nutrition), genetic, and biochemical factors during fetal, neonatal, and early childhood life that play a role in defining the offspring phenotype and as risk determinants for noncommunicable diseases. Professionally, Dr. Atkinson has and continues to serve on various grant review panels in Canada and Europe as well as expert and advisory panels struck by the National Academies of Sciences, Engineering, and Medicine (Food and Nutrition Board), the Office of Dietary Supplements of the National Institutes of Health or Health Canada that relate to development of the Dietary Reference Intakes (DRIs) and *Dietary Guidelines for Americans*. She is chair of the Board of Directors of the Maternal, Infant, Child and Youth Health Research Network (MICYRN) and co-lead of the MICYRN Canadian Birth Cohort Coalition to harmonize data from Canadian birth cohort studies. Her professional service and achievements in nutrition research have been recognized through receipt of many national awards including election as a fellow in the Canadian Academy of Health Sciences and the American Society for Nutrition, the Governor General of Canada's award of the Queen Elizabeth II Diamond Jubilee Medal, and an Honorary Doctor of Science from her alma mater, Western University.

Francesco Branca, Ph.D., is the director of the Department of Nutrition for Health and Development in the World Health Organization in Geneva. He graduated in medicine and surgery and specialized in diabetology and metabolic diseases at the Università Cattolica del Sacro Cuore, Roma. He obtained a Ph.D. in nutrition at Aberdeen University. He was a senior scientist at the Italian Food and Nutrition Research Institute, where he was responsible for the design and implementation of several studies on the effects of food and nutrients on human health at the different stages of the life cycle, and for the design, management, and evaluation of public health nutrition programs. He was president of the Federation of the European Nutrition Societies from 2003–2007.

Peter Clifton, Ph.D., is professor of nutrition at the University of South Australia and a research fellow at Baker International Diabetes Institute (IDI) Heart and Diabetes Institute. He is an internationally respected leader in the field of cardiovascular disease, nutrition, and health. To date, Dr. Clifton has contributed to informing scientific opinion through publication of 164 journal articles, more than 100 of these in the last 10 years, 6 book chapters, and many scientific presentations. Dr. Clifton actively contributes to the provision of scientific leadership to the food industry sector and has positively influenced the health of Australians through his high profile in publications such as the *Total Wellbeing Diet* while at Commonwealth Scientific and Industrial Research Organisation (CSIRO) and more recently the *Diabetes, Diet and Lifestyle Plan* (Penguin 2011).

Umi Fahmida, Ph.D., M.Sc., is the deputy director for programs at the Southeast Asian Ministers of Education Organization Regional Center for Food and Nutrition (SEAMEO RECFON) at the University of Indonesia, Jakarta. At SEAMEO RECFON, she performs research-teaching-consultancy activities in community nutrition. She also teaches the Nutrition Study Program for postgraduate students in the Faculty of Medicine at the University of Indonesia. She earned her bachelor's degree from the Faculty of Agriculture Technology, Bogor Agriculture University, and her M.Sc. in community nutrition and Ph.D. in nutrition from the Faculty of Medicine, University of Indonesia. She received a postdoctoral research award from the Scientific Programme Indonesia-Netherlands for her nutrigenomics/nutrigenetics study on the role of long-chain polyunsaturated fatty acids and iron on young child cognition. Her research interest is on the use of linear/goal programming to develop and evaluate food-based recommendations and the effects of nutrient and non-nutrient (psychosocial stimulation, gene) interactions on infant and child growth and development. Dr. Fahmida and her team have done extensive work on the use of linear/goal programming to develop and evaluate complementary feeding recommendations in Cambodia, Indonesia, Lao People's Democratic Republic, and Myanmar and advised postgraduate students from Cambodia, Indonesia, Malaysia, Myanmar, and the Philippines on this topic. She is also a member of the editorial board of the *Malaysian Journal of Nutrition*.

Susan Fairweather-Tait, Ph.D., is a professor at Norwich Medical School at the University of East Anglia (UEA). After she received her Ph.D. at King's College London (formerly Queen Elizabeth College), she worked in the food industry for a short while and then moved to the Institute of Food Research, Norwich, initially as a senior research scientist and later as head of the nutrition division and program leader for micronutrients. In 2006 she was offered a personal chair in the School of Medicine, Health Policy & Practice at UEA and moved to UEA in early 2007. Dr. Fairweather-Tait's research expertise is in micronutrients, in particular iron bioavailability and requirements for optimal health, using a combination of cell/in vitro models and human studies and working in collaboration with colleagues both nationally and internationally. Her current teaching activity is focused on undergraduate medical degree students (nutrition, diet and health, and preventive medicine) and postgraduate students. Her lectures include diet and bone health, nutritional anemias, and micronutrient requirements.

Rosalind Gibson, Ph.D., M.S.P.H., is an emerita professor in the Department of Human Nutrition, University of Otago, Dunedin, New Zealand. She has an M.S. in public health (nutrition) from the School of Public Health, University of California, Los Angeles, and a Ph.D. in nutrition from the University of London, United Kingdom. She has had a lifelong interest in international nutrition, initially working in the Ethio-Swedish Children's Nutrition Unit in Ethiopia for 3 years, and subsequently in collaborative research studies on micronutrients in Papua New Guinea, Guatemala, Ghana, Malawi, Zambia, and Ethiopia as well as Thailand, Mongolia, and more recently Cambodia, Northeastern Brazil, and Indonesia. Before joining the University of Otago, she was a faculty member in the Division of Applied Nutrition, University of Guelph. Dr. Gibson is a member of the International Zinc Nutrition Collaborative Group (IZiNCG), a fellow of the American Society of Nutrition, and a fellow of the Royal Society of New Zealand. She is the author of a standard reference text, *Principles of Nutritional Assessment*, published by Oxford University Press and regularly teaches short courses on this topic in Indonesia and Ethiopia, and formerly in Thailand and South Africa. She has been co-director of the World Health Organization Collaborating Centre for Nutrition in the Western Pacific Region in the department until 2017 and is the recipient of the McHenry Award by the Canadian Society of Nutritional Sciences, the Rank Prize from the British Nutrition Society, and the Kellogg International Prize by the American Society of Nutrition. Her research interests focus on etiology and impact of micronutrient deficiencies on growth, development, and health, and emphasize sustainable food-based strategies to combat micronutrient deficiencies.

Hasan Hutchinson, Ph.D., N.D., is the director general of the Office of Nutrition Policy and Promotion within the Health Products and Food Branch of Health Canada. As the focal point for public health nutrition within the federal government, the office strives to promote the nutritional health and well-being of Canadians. The office's main functions include dietary guidance, food and nutrition surveillance, research and data analysis, health promotion, and public health nutrition policy. Dr. Hutchinson is also the co-chair of the Federal/Provincial/Territorial Group on Nutrition and of the multisectoral Network on Healthy Eating. He serves on a number of nutrition-related committees at the World Health Organization and Pan American Health Organization and has served on a number of health-related committees at the Organisation for Economic Co-operation and Development and at the United Nations. He also served as chair of Canada's Sodium Working Group.

Janet King, Ph.D., R.D., is executive director of Children's Hospital Oakland Research Institute (CHORI) and professor of nutrition at the University of California, Berkeley, and Davis. Throughout a long and distinguished career, Dr. King has made substantive contributions to the body of human nutrition research, application, and policy development. In recognition of her national and international reputation, she was elected to the National Academy of Medicine in 1994, and in 2007, she was inducted into the U.S. Department of Agriculture (USDA) Research Hall of Fame. She directed the USDA Western Human Nutrition Research Center at the University of California, Davis (1995–2002) and chaired the Department of Nutritional Sciences, University of California, Berkeley (1988–1994). Dr. King's research focuses on metabolic adjustments to changes in nutrient intakes in humans; she is especially interested in metabolism and nutrient utilization of pregnant and lactating women. Dr. King's impact on the field of human nutrition extends well beyond her research accomplishments. For example, she chaired the USDA/U.S. Department of Health and Human Services (HHS) Dietary Guidelines Advisory Committee. The committee's work resulted in the publication of the *Dietary Guidelines for Americans 2005* that had a significant impact on what Americans eat. When Dr. King was the chair of the Institute of Medicine's Food and Nutrition Board in 1994, the paradigm for the then new Dietary Reference Intakes was established. She recently chaired a United Nations University, Food and Agriculture Organization, World Health Organization Joint Committee on Dietary Harmonization and is a member of the United Nations International Consultative Group on Zinc.

Anura Kurpad, M.D., Ph.D., is a professor and the head of physiology and nutrition at St John's Medical College, Bangalore, India, and was the Founding Dean of St John's Research Institute, Bangalore, India. He is presently the head of the first International Atomic Energy Agency Collaborating Centre on Nutrition, located at St John's, and is the past-president of the Nutrition Society of India. He is a fellow of the National Academy of Medical Sciences, fellow of the International Union of Nutritional Sciences, and Margdarshi fellow of the Wellcome Trust-DBT India Alliance. He has published 350 papers, and is co-author of the Asian Edition of *Guyton's Textbook of Physiology*, co-editor of the *Asia Pacific Journal of Clinical Nutrition*, and associate editor of the *European Journal of Clinical Nutrition*. He is the chairman of the Scientific Advisory Group of the Nutrition Division of the Indian Council of Medical Research (ICMR); Scientific Advisory Committee of the National Institute of Nutrition; ICMR Expert Committee on Tolerable Upper Limits of Nutrients; ICMR Task Force on Improving Health and Nutritional Status of Vulnerable Segments of the Population; ICMR Task Force on Indian Comprehensive Health and

Nutrition Survey; the Protein Quality Group at the Nevin Scrimshaw International Nutrition Foundation; and the Ethics Committee of the National Institute of Mental Health and Neurosciences, Bangalore.

Anna Lartey, Ph.D., M.Sc., is the president of the International Union of Nutritional Sciences (2013–2017) and director of nutrition at the Food and Agriculture Organization of the United Nations, Rome, Italy (October 2013–present). She was a professor of nutrition at the University of Ghana (1986–2013). Dr. Lartey attended the University of California, Davis, as a Fulbright student and received her Ph.D. in international nutrition. She received her M.Sc. and B.Sc. degrees from the University of Guelph, and the University of Ottawa, Canada. Subsequent to this she worked as a researcher in sub-Saharan Africa for 27 years. Her research focused on maternal child nutrition. She has received several awards; among these are the University of Ghana's "Best Researcher Award for 2004"; the International Development Research Center (IDRC, Canada) Research Chair in Nutrition for Health and Socioeconomic Development in sub-Saharan Africa (2009–2014); African Nutrition Society award (2014) for contribution to nutrition research and capacity building; Ghana Women of Excellence Award (2012) for contribution to science and nutrition research in Ghana; "Yokama" (Ideal Woman) from the Manya Krobo Traditional Council for contribution to the development of the District; and she is the recipient of the Sight and Life Nutrition Leadership Award for 2014. During her tenure as International Union of Nutritional Sciences president, the statues and rules of the organization have been completely rewritten to bring them in line with practices of a modern scientific society.

Joseph Lau, M.D., is professor in the Center for Evidence-based Medicine within the School of Public Health and codirector of the Agency for Healthcare Research and Quality (AHRQ) designated Evidence-based Practice Center (EPC) at Brown University. Prior to his current position, he was professor of medicine and professor of clinical and translational science at the Institute for Clinical Research and Health Policy Studies at Tufts Medical Center. He directed the Tufts EPC from 1997 until 2012 and led the production of more than 80 evidence reports, technology assessments, and comparative effectiveness reviews under contract with the AHRQ. He has served as a member of a Food and Drug Administration advisory committee, and as a member of a Food and Agriculture Organization/World Health Organization workshop. He served as a member on two Institute of Medicine (IOM) committees including the framework to evaluate the safety of dietary supplements and standards for clinical practice guidelines. He received his M.D. from Tufts University School of Medicine and completed a fellowship in clinical decision making and medical computer science at the New England Medical Center.

Catherine Leclercq, Ph.D., is a nutritionist and expert of food consumption studies and dietary assessment. She was previously a senior researcher at the Italian Agricultural Research Council. She served for more than 10 years as a member of a panel of the European Food Safety Authority and on Food and Agriculture Organization/World Health Organization (FAO/WHO) expert committees as an expert of dietary exposure to food chemicals. She joined the Nutrition Division (ESN) at the Headquarters of the Food and Agriculture Organization of the United Nations in August 2013. Dr. Leclercq is leading the development of a new tool FAO/WHO GIFT (FAO/WHO Global Individual Food consumption data Tool), which is aimed at dramatically enhancing the use of existing individual food consumption data for nutrition and food safety purposes worldwide. This tool will answer key information needs of policy makers at country, regional, and global levels in the field of nutrition and food safety.

Amanda MacFarlane, Ph.D., is a research scientist in the Nutrition Research Division, Food Directorate, Health Canada. She received her Ph.D. in 2004 in Biochemistry in the lab of Dr. Fraser Scott from the University of Ottawa. Her Ph.D. work focused on defining the mechanism by which diet promotes autoimmune diabetes via an abnormal immune response in the gut for which she won the 2003 Ron Oelbaum Award for an Outstanding Canadian Research Scientist under the age of 35 from the Juvenile Diabetes Research Foundation. She did her postdoctoral research in the lab of Dr. Patrick Stover in the Division of Nutritional Sciences at Cornell University where she examined the effect of altered folate metabolism on genome stability and gene expression in colon cancer. She joined Health Canada as a research scientist in 2008. Her research examines the biochemical, genetic, and epigenetic mechanisms that underlie relationships between folic acid and chronic disease with a focus on cancer. In addition, she uses biochemical and molecular genetics approaches to study the effect of maternal dietary folate status during pregnancy on disease susceptibility in the offspring.

Christophe Matthys, Ph.D., is an assistant professor in human nutrition at the Katholieke Universiteit Leuven, Belgium, and Scientific Coordinator of the clinical nutrition unit of the University Hospital Leuven, Belgium. Dr. Matthys has international research experience in the different domains of human nutrition (e.g., food consumption and nutrition surveys, nutrition policy and public health nutrition, nutritional epidemiology, experimental studies in nutritional epidemiology, food safety). He is an active member of the Belgian Nutrition Society and the European Nutrition Leadership Platform. He is currently a member of the Scientific Committee of the Belgian Federal Agency for the Safety of the Food Chain.

Helle Margrete Meltzer, Ph.D., is the research director of the Norwegian Institute of Public Health. She has many years of experience in food, nutrition, and health research. In recent years, she has been particularly interested in looking at nutrition in a larger perspective and believes that nutritionists' responsibility should not stop at knowledge-based dietary advice based on health, but also help solve the issues of what is a sustainable future. She is a member of the National Council for Nutrition, where she currently works specifically with sustainability issues. Dr. Meltzer received her Ph.D. in nutrition from the University of Oslo.

Suzanne Murphy, Ph.D., R.D., is a researcher emerita at the University of Hawaii Cancer Center in Honolulu. Dr. Murphy's research interests are both national and international, and include dietary assessment methodology, food and supplement composition databases, development and use of nutrient standards, and the nutritional epidemiology of chronic diseases. Dr. Murphy was elected treasurer of the International Union of Nutritional Sciences (IUNS) for two terms and co-chaired two IUNS task forces: the International Network of Food Data Systems (INFOODS) and Dietary Quality Indicators. She has served on several Institute of Medicine panels including the Subcommittee on Interpretation and Uses of Dietary Reference Intakes (as chair then member); the Subcommittee on Upper Safe Reference Levels of Nutrients (as member), and the Panel on Calcium and Related Nutrients (as member). She chaired the Committee to Review the WIC Food Packages and the Committee to Review Child and Adult Care Food Programs, and was a member of the Committee to Review the School Meals Programs. She is a member of the National Academy of Medicine and a fellow of the American Society for Nutrition. Dr. Murphy has received the Excellence in Dietary Guidance Award from the American Public Health Association, the Monsen Award for Outstanding Research Literature from the Academy of Nutrition and Dietetics, the Lifetime Achievement Award from the Steering Committee of the National Nutrient Databank Conference, and the Elvehjem Award for Public Service in Nutrition from the American Society for Nutrition. Dr. Murphy earned an M.S. in molecular biology from San Francisco State University and a Ph.D. degree in nutrition from the University of California, Berkeley.

John Muyonga, Ph.D., is a professor in the Department of Food Technology and Human Nutrition at Makerere University, Uganda, and current dean of the School of Food Technology, Nutrition, and Bioengineering. He is widely published and cited in the fields of food science and nutrition. His research covers aspects of nutritional and nutraceutical properties of understudied foods, food processing, and processing waste valorization. He has also worked on determination of nutrition and food security status in different areas in Uganda, as well as on aspects of management of malnutrition. As university leader, he has been at the forefront of promoting research application.

Chizuru Nishida, Ph.D., is the coordinator of the Nutrition Policy and Scientific Advice Unit (NPU) in the Department of Nutrition for Health and Development (NHD) at the World Health Organization Headquarters (WHO/HQ) in Geneva. Her career in WHO began in 1984 in the Maternal and Child Health Programme in the WHO/HQ where she worked on WHO's research project on infant and young child feeding and rearing practices developed as part of the Joint United Nations Children's Fund/WHO Nutrition Support Programme (JNSP). She also worked in the WHO Regional Office for the Western Pacific and on several country office programmes. In 1990, she moved back to WHO/HQ to serve as the WHO secretariat for the 1992 International Conference on Nutrition (ICN), which adopted the World Declaration and Plan of Action for Nutrition, a blueprint for member states in developing their nutrition policies and action plans. In 2014, she also served as a WHO secretariat of the 2nd International Conference on Nutrition (ICN2) which adopted the Rome Declaration on Nutrition and Framework for Action and led to the proclamation of the Decade of Action on Nutrition (2016–2025) by the United Nations General Assembly in April 2016. As the coordinator of NPU, currently she leads the work on: (1) development, updating, and dissemination of science-based guidelines and policy actions for preventing obesity and diet-related noncommunicable diseases; and (2) provision of guidance and support to the regions and countries in translating WHO guidelines into policy and program interventions through developing operational tools (including nutrient profile models and nutrition labeling) and providing capacity building training to address all forms of malnutrition throughout the life course. She also represents WHO at several Codex committees, particularly those related to nutrition and food labeling.

Caryl Nowson, Ph.D., is a professor of nutrition and aging at Deakin University's School of Exercise and Nutrition. She teaches at the undergraduate and postgraduate level and also supervises higher-degree students. Dr. Nowson is a member of the Centre for Physical Activity and Nutrition Research (C-PAN) and has a specific focus on reducing risk of cardiovascular disease and osteoporosis through preventive strategies that extend throughout the life span. Dr. Nowson's research primarily centers on nutrition related to hypertension and bone health. In addition to conducting a range of dietary and lifestyle intervention studies, she has recently focused on informing and changing policy to reduce risk of chronic disease, specifically cardiovascular disease and osteoporosis.

James Ntambi, Ph.D., received his B.S. and M.S. degrees in biochemistry and chemistry from Makerere University in Kampala, Uganda, and his Ph.D. degree in biochemistry and molecular biology from the Johns Hopkins University School of Medicine in Baltimore, Maryland. He did his graduate and postdoctoral work at the Johns Hopkins University School of Medicine in the laboratories of Drs. Paul T. Englund and M. Daniel Lane, respectively, where he started his work on the molecular biology of parasites and the regulation of genes of lipid metabolism. Dr. Ntambi has made distinguished contributions to the field of nutritional biochemistry, and his pioneering work on the genetic regulation of the stearoyl-coenzyme A desaturase has recently led to many new insights into the importance of this enzyme in metabolism and in disease states, such as obesity, diabetes, atherosclerosis, inflammation, and cancer. His pioneering work will help explain the complex aspects of the "metabolic syndrome" and to advance our understanding of nutrient–gene interactions. Dr. Ntambi has published more than 150 peer-reviewed scientific papers and is also involved in international research and teaching efforts, including student and faculty exchange programs between Makerere University and the University of Wisconsin–Madison. He has received numerous awards, including the Osborne and Mendel Award, the Steenbock Career Development Award, the Fogarty International Biomedical Research Award, the Fulbright Research Award, the Arthur J. Maurer Extra Mile Award, the Excellence in International Activities Award, the Distinguished Chancellor's Teaching Award, and the American Society for Biochemistry and Molecular Biology Award for Exemplary Contributions to Education. Dr. Ntambi serves in National Institutes of Health (NIH) study sections and is a member of the NIH/National Institute on Alcohol Abuse and Alcoholism Board of Scientific Counselors. He is also a member of the Institute of Medicine Food and Nutrition Board of the National Academies of Sciences, Engineering, and Medicine. He has been invited to present seminars on obesity and diabetes research at conferences in the United States and other countries, serves on numerous scientific committees, and is an advisor to government agencies. He has recently been inducted into the Uganda National Academy of Sciences.

Hee Young Paik, Sc.D., currently serves as the director of the Center for Gendered Innovations Research, Korea Federation of Women's Science and Technology Associations (KOFWST), in Korea and professor emerita of Seoul National University. Dr. Paik received a doctor of science in nutrition from the Harvard School of Public Health in Boston, Massachusetts. After receiving her doctoral degree, she worked as a faculty member at Sookmyung Women's University and then at Seoul National University in Korea until February 2016. She worked in various professional organizations serving various roles including president of the Korean Home Economics Association in 2013, the Korean Nutrition Society in 2015, and the Korea Federation of Women's Science and Technology Associations from 2014 to 2016. She was the chair of the Korean Dietary Reference Intakes Committee from 2002 to 2005, when the Dietary Reference Intakes for Koreans were newly developed in Korea. She was a member of the International Union of Nutritional Sciences Council from 2005 to 2009, and received several honors including Excellent Research Awards in Science (2005), National Honor for High Achievements in Science (2008), and Asia-Pacific Clinical Nutrition Award (2009), and the Blue Ribbon National Medal for Public Service (2012). Dr. Paik served as the minister of gender equality and family, Republic of Korea, 2009–2011.

Ann Prentice, O.B.E., Ph.D., D.U.S., Hon.F.R.C.P.C.H., Hon.F.N.S., F.Med. Sci., F.Af.N., F.R.S.B., is the director at Medical Research Council Elsie Widdowson Laboratory (EWL), as well as head of the Nutrition and Bone Health Group. Her research focuses on nutrient requirements for bone health, encompassing the nutritional problems of both affluent and developing societies. She is currently involved in projects studying pregnant and lactating women, children, adolescents, and older people in the United Kingdom, West Africa, Bangladesh, South Africa, and China. Dr. Prentice is chair of the United Kingdom Scientific Advisory Committee on Nutrition and a member of a number of other advisory committees. She is a fellow of the Academy of Medical Science and the Society of Biology; an honorary fellow of the Royal College of Paediatrics and Child Health; an honorary professor of the University of Witwatersrand, South Africa, and Shenyang Medical College, China; and a visiting professor of nutritional science at the University of Southampton. Dr. Prentice was awarded the British Nutrition Foundation Prize in 2011; the Laureate de Le Prix Scientifique, Institut Candia, France, in 1998; the Robert and Edna Langholz Award for International Nutrition in 2004; and an honorary doctorate from the University of Surrey in 2014. She was president of the Nutrition Society between 2004 and 2007 and appointed an OBE in the Birthday Honours List 2006.

Hildegard Przyrembel, M.D., Ph.D., started her career at the University Children's Hospital Ulm working on a project financed by the German Society for Research on the amino acid requirement of premature infants, combining analytical laboratory work with a clinical education in pediatrics, with special emphasis on inborn errors of metabolism. After moving to the University Children's Hospital Düsseldorf for the continuation of her specialization in pediatrics, Dr. Przyrembel was, in addition, head of the laboratory for inborn errors of metabolism. This work, in cooperation with the metabolic laboratories of the Hammersmith Hospital, London, and the University Children's Hospital in Utrecht, led to the discovery and definition of two new inborn errors of lysine metabolism. This was also the basis of her inaugural dissertation in 1979. In 1980, Dr. Przyrembel moved to the University Children's Hospital Rotterdam and the Department of Cell Biology and Clinical Genetics of the Erasmus-University, Rotterdam, to become head of the Unit for Metabolic Disorders and of the Metabolic Laboratory. In cooperation with the Department of Biochemistry, the emphasis of her work shifted to defects in fatty acid oxidation and of the mitochondrial respiratory chain and their accessability to therapeutic measures. During this period she spent 3 months at the John F. Kennedy Child Development Center in Denver, Colorado. She was a member of the Dutch Guidance Committee for the Treatment of Phenylketonuria and contributed chapters to Dutch textbooks on pediatrics and medical genetics. In 1990, Dr. Przyrembel accepted a position in the Unit Nutrition in Medicine at the Federal Institute of Health at Berlin. This included analytical laboratory work, namely the analysis of the composition of nonprotein nitrogen in infant formula. She worked predominantly as a consultant in infant and child nutrition and dietetic therapy, both on national and international panels. Since the foundation of the Federal Institute for Risk Assessment in November 2002, Dr. Przyrembel's tasks have been on the assessment of both benefits and risks in connection with dietary habits, including breastfeeding, and connected with the use of ingredients, nutrients, whole foods, and with residues (if the latter occur in human milk or foods for infants and children). In 2000, Dr. Przyrembel started as an expert and rapporteur (biotin, calcium, protein, and carbohydrates in infant formula) in the working groups on upper levels of vitamins and minerals, on infant formula composition, and on food additives (nutrient compounds) of the Scientific Committee on Food of the European Commission. Dr. Przyrembel was appointed a member of the Scientific Panel on Nutrition, Dietetic Foods, and Allergy of the European Food Safety Authority (EFSA) in May 2003. Recent and actual tasks for EFSA include setting nutrient reference values, including upper levels for minerals and vitamins; safety of new ingredients in infant formula; safety of trans fatty acids; safety and benefits of fish consumption; and assessment of the scientific justification of claims in connection with nutrients/foods and nutritional effects of foods consisting of or derived from genetically modified organisms (contribution to >400 EFSA Opinions).

Kostas Stamoulis, Ph.D., is currently the assistant director-general a.i. of the Economic and Social Development Department at the Food and Agriculture Organization (FAO) of the United Nations. He served as director, strategic programme leader, Food Security and Nutrition, in FAO. He led through 2015 the design and provided strategic guidance of FAO's Strategic Programme on Food Security and Nutrition, which cuts across several disciplines and geographical regions. Between 2008 and 2015 he was the director of the Agricultural Development Economics Division (ESA) of FAO. ESA carries out the bulk of analytical and evidence-based policy work of FAO with about 150 staff members. From 2007 to 2015 he was the secretary of the Committee on World Food Security and played a key role in the reform of the committee. Since joining FAO he has held progressively responsible technical and management positions. Before joining FAO in 1989, he was assistant professor of agricultural economics at the University of Illinois at Urbana-Champaign. From 1985 to 1987 he was a postdoctoral fellow at the University of California, Berkeley. His work includes issues related to the role of agriculture in rural development and rural poverty reduction in developing countries; the impact of changes in food systems on smallholder farmers and on rural poverty; the linkages between the agricultural sector and the rural nonfarm economy; and the integration of food security and nutrition in sectorial policies and programs. He has also carried out work on the assessment of the role of macroeconomic and exchange-rate policies on agriculture and the rural sector and the interdependence between exchange rates and financial and commodity markets. He has published a large number of papers, articles, books, and monographs on a variety of subjects. He holds a degree in economics from the Economics University of Athens (Greece), a master's degree in agricultural economics from the University of Georgia (USA), and a Ph.D. in agricultural and resource economics from the University of California, Berkeley.

Patrick J. Stover, Ph.D., is a professor and the director of the Division of Nutritional Sciences at Cornell University. He is also director of the United Nations Food and Nutrition Program for Human and Social Development at Cornell University and vice president elect of the American Society for Nutritional Sciences. Dr. Stover's research interests focus on the biochemical, genetic, and epigenetic mechanisms that underlie the relationships between folic acid and human pathologies including neural tube defects and other developmental anomalies, cardiovascular disease, and cancer. Specific interests include the regulation of folate-mediated one-carbon metabolism and cellular methylation reactions, molecular basis of the fetal origins hypothesis, development of mouse models to elucidate mechanisms of folate-related pathologies, and translational control of gene expression by ferritin. In 1976, he received the Presidential Early Career Award for Scientists and

Engineers, the highest honor bestowed by the U.S. government on outstanding scientists and engineers beginning their independent careers. He received the ERL Stokstad Award in Nutritional Biochemistry from the American Society for Nutritional Sciences in 1999 and has been selected as an Outstanding Educator four times by Cornell Merrill Presidential Scholars.

Emorn Udomkesmalee, Ph.D., is the senior advisor and former director of the Institute of Nutrition, Mahidol University, Thailand. She holds a current position of adjunct associate professor in the Department of International Health, Bloomberg School of Public Health, Johns Hopkins University. Her research interests include micronutrient assessment, bioavailability, and metabolism; micronutrient interaction especially of vitamin A and zinc or iron and zinc; and micronutrient and immune function. She is currently a member of several international bodies and international committees: the Country Network of the Scaling Up Nutrition Movement; World Health Organization Nutrition Guidance Expert Advisory Group on Micronutrients; the International Zinc Nutrition Consultative Group; Steering Committee of the Micronutrient Forum; the International Union of Nutritional Sciences Council; the Global Alliance for Improved Nutrition Partnership Council; International Food Policy Research Institute Strategic Advisory Council; the International Obesity Task Force Scientific Advisory Council; and the Culinary Institute of America's Worlds of Healthy Flavors Scientific and Public Health Advisory Committee, as well as the Scientific Director of International Life Sciences Institute South East Asia Region.

Hans Verhagen, Ph.D., is the head of the European Food Safety Authority's (EFSA's) Risk Assessment and Scientific Assistance Department, which performs risk assessments on general health and safety issues in biological hazards, chemical contaminants, plant health, animal health and welfare, and provides support on data collection, emerging risks, exposure assessment, and risk assessment methodologies. Before EFSA he worked at the Rijkinstitut voor Volksgezondheid en Milieu (Netherlands National Institute for Public Health and the Environment) and Toegepast Natuurweten Schappelijk Onderzoek (Netherlands Organisation for Applied Scientific Research), in Unilever Research and at the Universities of Maastricht and Nijmegen (Netherlands). He was member of EFSA's Panel on Dietetic Products, Nutrition and Allergies from 2006 to 2015. He is a board-certified toxicologist and nutritionist and a visiting professor at the University of Ulster in Northern Ireland from 2009.

George Wells, Ph.D., is the director of the Cardiovascular Research Methods Centre at the University of Ottawa Heart Institute and a professor in the School of Epidemiology, Public Health and Preventive Medicine, at the University of Ottawa. Also at the University of Ottawa, he serves as a professor in the Department of Medicine and senior scientist affiliate at the Ottawa Hospital Research Institute. Dr. Wells has worked extensively with national and international government and nongovernment research organizations, as well as private pharmaceutical and biotechnology industries. He has been on the executive and steering committees of national and international research programs as well as on committees with the following focus: external safety and efficacy monitoring, scientific grant review, editorial, and scientific advisory. He is currently an associate editor of the *Journal of Clinical Epidemiology* and on the Editorial Committee for the *Canadian Medical Association Journal*. Dr. Wells received the University of Ottawa Excellence in Research Award in 2014 and the Canadian Society for Clinical Investigation Distinguished Scientist Award in 2007.